Leadership and Management in Nursing Test Success

Ruth A. Wittmann-Price, PhD, RN, CNS, CNE, is chairperson and professor at Francis Marion University Department of Nursing in South Carolina. Ruth has been an obstetrical/women's health nurse for 35 years. She received her AAS and BSN degrees from Felician College in Lodi, NJ (1978, 1981), and her MS as a perinatal CNS from Columbia University, NY (1983). Ruth completed her PhD at Widener University, Chester, PA (2006), and was awarded the Dean's Award for Excellence. She developed a mid-range nursing theory, "Emancipated Decision-Making in Women's Health Care." Besides continuing her research about decisional science, she studies developmental outcomes of preterm infants. She has also been the director of nursing research for Hahnemann University Hospital (2007–2010) and oversees all evidence-based practice projects for nursing. Hahnemann University Hospital was awarded initial Magnet status (American Nurses Credentialing Center) in December 2009. Ruth has taught all levels of nursing students over the past 15 years (AAS, BSN, MSN, and DNP) and completed an international service learning trip (2007) to rural Mexico with undergraduate nursing and physician assistant students. She was the coordinator for the nurse educator track in the DrNP program at Drexel University in Philadelphia (2007–2010) and sits on four dissertation committees. Ruth is coeditor and chapter contributor of eight books, *Nursing Education: Foundations for Practice Excellence* (2007) (AJN Book of the Year Award winner 2007); *Certified Nurse Examination (CNE) Review Manual* (2012) (and the Second Edition [2013]); *NCLEX-RN® EXCEL Test Success Through Unfolding Case Study Review* (2010); *Maternal-Child Nursing Test Success: An Unfolding Case Study Review* (2012); *Fundamentals of Nursing Test Success: An Unfolding Case Study Review* (2013); *Nursing Concept Care Maps for Safe Patient Care* (2013); and *Community Health Nursing Test Success* (2013). She has published the chapter "The Newborn at Risk" in *Maternal-Child Nursing Care: Optimizing Outcomes for Mothers, Children, and Families*, a section in *Giving Through Teaching: How Nurse Educators Are Changing the World*, and over 20 journal articles.

Frances H. Cornelius, PhD, MSN, RN-BC, CNE, is associate clinical professor, chair of the MSN Advanced Practice Role Department and coordinator of informatics projects at Drexel University, College of Nursing and Health Professions. Fran has taught nursing since 1991, at several schools of nursing. She taught community health at Madonna University (Livonia, MI), Oakland (MI) University, University of Pittsburgh (PA), and Holy Family College (Philadelphia, PA). Fran taught adult health and gerontology at Widener University School of Nursing until 1997, when she began teaching at Drexel. In 2003, she was a Fellow at the Biomedical Library of Medicine. She is a certified nurse informaticist and has been the recipient of several grants. She has collaborated on the development of mobile applications as coordinator of informatics projects, including the Patient Assessment and Care Plan Development (PACPD) tool, which is a PDA tool with a Web-based companion, and Gerontology Reasoning Informatics Programs (the GRIP project). She is the coeditor (with Mary Gallagher Gordon) and chapter contributor of *PDA Connections*, an innovative textbook designed to teach health care professionals how to use mobile devices for point-of-care access of information. She is a coauthor of *Maternal-Child Nursing Test Success: An Unfolding Case Study Review* (2012); *Fundamentals of Nursing Test Success: An Unfolding Case Study Review* (2013); *Medical-Surgical Nursing Test Success: An Unfolding Case Study Review* (2013); and *Community Health Nursing Test Success: An Unfolding Case Study Review* (2013). She has written six book chapters and has published 19 journal articles on her work. She has been invited to deliver 26 presentations and has delivered more than 50 peer-reviewed presentations mostly in the United States, but also in Spain, Canada, and Korea. She is a member of the American Informatics Association, the American Nursing Informatics Association, the American Nurses Association, and the Pennsylvania State Nurses Association.

Leadership and Management in Nursing Test Success: An Unfolding Case Study Review

Ruth A. Wittmann-Price, PhD, RN, CNS, CNE
Frances H. Cornelius, PhD, MSN, RN-BC, CNE

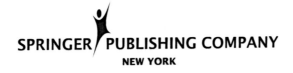

SPRINGER PUBLISHING COMPANY
NEW YORK

Springer Publishing Company, LLC
11 West 42nd Street
New York, NY 10036
www.springerpub.com

Acquisitions Editor: Margaret Zuccarini
Composition: S4Carlisle Publishing Services

ISBN: 978-0-8261-1038-1
E-book ISBN: 978-0-8261-1039-8
eResources ISBN: 978-0-8261-9424-4

A list of eResources is available from www.springerpub.com/wittmann-price-ancillaries

13 14 15 / 5 4 3 2 1

Library of Congress Cataloging-in-Publication Data
Wittmann-Price, Ruth A.
Leadership and management in nursing test success : an unfolding case study review / Ruth A. Wittmann-Price, Frances H. Cornelius.
    p. ; cm.
Includes bibliographical references and index.
ISBN 978-0-8261-1038-1 — ISBN 0-8261-1038-X — ISBN 978-0-8261-1039-8 (e-book)
I. Cornelius, Frances H.   II. Title.
[DNLM: 1. Leadership—Problems and Exercises. 2. Nursing Care—Problems and Exercises. 3. Nursing Process—Problems and Exercises. 4. Nursing, Supervisory—Problems and Exercises. WY 18.2]
RT55
610.73076—dc23
                                                                                        2013008723

Printed in the United States of America by Bradford & Bigelow.

This book is dedicated to the loving memory of my brother Kenny.
Ruth A. Wittmann-Price

Contents

Preface

Nurses as leaders at the bedside, within health care systems, and as a part of health care teams are becoming more and more important. Nurses are the health care professionals that are there 24/7; they are the first line of defense for patient, family, and community care and safety. They advocate for patients, families, and communities and understand their needs better than anyone else. Leadership in nursing is becoming a much overused term to encompass multiple skills. This book breaks down those skill sets and allows the learners of nursing leadership to practice those skills in a cognitive way by placing themselves into simulated unfolding case studies.

The case studies can be used in any number of creative and innovative ways, such as using the embedded questions to test your knowledge acquisition of the content or using the Internet links to further develop understanding of a subject. **A list of these web links and resources is available from www.springerpub. com/wittmann-price-ancillaries.** Other ways that these unfolding case study books have been used with great success are as interactive adjunct material to leadership courses and self-study modules for make-up clinical experiences. The obvious use of this book is for NCLEX-RN® practice to build confidence and self-efficacy in leadership skills, which are a necessary part of standardized testing and the licensure exam.

We hope you enjoy this book as you have the other unfolding case study books in this series and use it to enhance your leadership skills. We know that this book is more engaging than a traditional question-and-answer book and provides the up-to-date Internet links that learners today use during clinical practice to enhance their decision-making ability in a leadership role.

Ruth A. Wittmann-Price, PhD, RN, CNS, CNE
Frances H. Cornelius, PhD, MSN, RN-BC, CNE

Acknowledgments

Thank you, Margaret Zuccarini, for being an inspiring nursing editor, and to Linda Wilson, RN, PhD, CPAN, CAPA, BC, CNE, CHSE, for sharing her expansive knowledge about electronic health records and simulation.

Nursing Test Success

With Ruth A. Wittmann-Price as Series Editor

Maternal-Child Nursing Test Success:
An Unfolding Case Study Review
Ruth A. Wittmann-Price, PhD, RN, CNS, CNE,
and Frances H. Cornelius, PhD, MSN, RN-BC, CNE

Fundamentals of Nursing Test Success:
An Unfolding Case Study Review
Ruth A. Wittmann-Price, PhD, RN, CNS, CNE,
and Frances H. Cornelius, PhD, MSN, RN-BC, CNE

Community Health Nursing Test Success:
An Unfolding Case Study Review
Frances H. Cornelius, PhD, MSN, RN-BC, CNE,
and Ruth A. Wittmann-Price, PhD, RN, CNS, CNE

Medical-Surgical Nursing Test Success:
An Unfolding Case Study Review
Karen K. Gittings, DNP, RN, CNE, Alumnus CCRN, Rhonda M. Brogdon,
DNP, MSN, MBA, RN, and Frances H. Cornelius, PhD, MSN, RN-BC, CNE

Leadership and Management in Nursing Test Success:
An Unfolding Case Study Review
Ruth A. Wittmann-Price, PhD, RN, CNS, CNE,
and Frances H. Cornelius, PhD, MSN, RN-BC, CNE

Leadership and Management in Nursing Test Success

1

Understanding the Complexity
of Leadership in Nursing

/

Unfolding Case Study #1 ▪ Beyonce and Jacob

Beyonce and Jacob are in their final semester of nursing education and are taking
a four-credit leadership course. There is a practicum to the course, so for 3 hours
a week they will have a chance to do some leadership activities. On the first day
of leadership class, after they review the syllabus, the nurse educator asks them
to identify the type of leader they believe they will be in their upcoming careers.
The learner's in the class have all been students for over 2 years and never really
envisioned themselves in leadership roles.

Exercise 1-1: *Multiple-choice question*
All nurses are leaders in patient health care primarily because they:
    A. Have the most education
    B. Administrate hospitals
    C. Know the patient the best
    D. Are with the patient the longest

The nurse educator explains that leadership and management are two different
things. Leaders are inspirational while managers plan and organize. Beyonce and
Jacob work on a fill-in exercise together.

Exercise 1-2: *Fill-in*
Place an "L" for leader and an "M" for manager beside the traits listed below:
    _____ Change agent
    _____ Future oriented
    _____ Time oriented
    _____ Visionary
    _____ Organizes
    _____ Budgets
    _____ Motivates
    _____ Consistency

Answers to this chapter begin on page 11.   **1**

During the first class, the nurse educator describes different leadership theories. Two of the more popular leadership theories today are *transactional* and *transformative*. Transactional leaders take care of their employees' needs while transformational leaders work alongside their employees.

Exercise 1-3: *Select all that apply*

Select the practices that are attributed to a transformational leader:

      ❑ Challenges the status quo

      ❑ Enforces changes

      ❑ Rewards employees who meet goals

      ❑ Motivates and inspires

      ❑ Empowers others

      ❑ Communicates down the organizational channels

Jacob asks the nurse educator if he would explain the other terms the leadership book uses to describe leaders. Dr. Bennett, the nurse educator, agrees that there are many theories and terms to describe leaders as well as leadership theories.

Exercise 1-4: *Matching*

Match the term in Column A to the description in Column B.

Column A	Column B
A. Autocratic	_____ Group makes the decisions, not the leader
B. Democratic	_____ Focuses on visions and values
C. Great-man theory	_____ Equally considers group opinion
D. Laissez-faire	_____ Characteristics that enable the leader
E. Situational leaders	_____ Born with an ability to lead others
F. Trait leaders	_____ Leader makes all the decisions
G. Transactional	_____ Traditional leadership style
H. Transformational	_____ An event determines the leader

Dr. Bennett provides further examples of *autocratic, democratic,* and *laissez-faire* leadership since these are traditional methods of describing leaders.

    e   **eResource 1-1:** Dr. Bennett shows the class brief videos regarding leadership:
        ■ *Leadership Styles:* http://goo.gl/001ns
        ■ *Inspirational Leader Versus Good Leader—What's the Difference?* http://goo.gl/dQ1AD

Beyonce, Jacob, and the rest of the senior learners use their automatic response system or clickers to answer the following questions.

Answers to this chapter begin on page 11.

Exercise 1-5: *Multiple-choice question*

A nurse requests a schedule change due to a family issue. The nurse manager states, "Find someone to switch with you." The nurse manager is demonstrating what type of leadership style?

A. Autocratic

B. Democratic

C. Laissez-faire

D. Transformational

Exercise 1-6: *Multiple-choice question*

A nurse requests a schedule change due to a family issue. The nurse manager states, "You cannot change the schedule without going through the staffing office." The nurse manager is demonstrating what type of leadership style?

A. Autocratic

B. Democratic

C. Laissez-faire

D. Transformational

Exercise 1-7: *Multiple-choice question*

A nurse requests a schedule change due to a family issue. The nurse manager states, "Let's develop a system to be proactive for all the staff when things like this happen." The nurse manager is demonstrating what type of leadership style?

A. Autocratic

B. Democratic

C. Laissez-faire

D. Transformational

 eResource 1-2: To test her understanding of leadership concepts, Beyonce completes *Distinguishing Leadership and Management Activities:* http://goo.gl/lJ6FU

Exercise 1-8: *Multiple-choice question*

A nurse requests a schedule change due to a family issue. The nurse manager states, "If you can't come in, we will figure it out." The nurse manager is demonstrating what type of leadership style?

A. Autocratic

B. Democratic

C. Laissez-faire

D. Transformational

Beyonce asks Dr. Bennett to further explain other types of leadership theories, not just transactional and transformational. Dr. Bennett explains that each leadership theory contains three factors that interact: the leaders, the followers, and the work environment.

Answers to this chapter begin on page 11.

Many theories concentrate on what motivates the followers to produce positive outcomes in the environment, which is sometimes referred to as the organization (Figure 1-1).

Figure 1-1: Three Factors in Leadership Theory

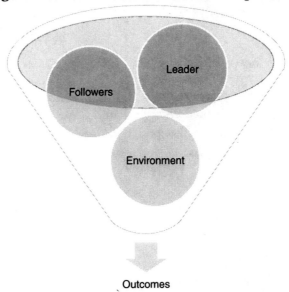

Dr. Bennett does tell the learners that leadership styles and theories are interwoven, so although it may seem confusing at first, they will notice that a leadership theory will identify the leadership style that works best within that theory.

 eResource 1-3: The instructor has the class take a leadership style test to provide students an opportunity to reflect upon their own leadership style: http://goo.gl/Pnx6X

An example is that a transformational leader would not work well in a hierarchical theory setting.

Exercise 1-9: *Matching*
Match the theory in Column A with the key points of the theory in Column B.

Column A	Column B
A. Trait theory	_____ Good outcomes motivate people
B. Style theory	_____ Physiological needs must be taken care of first
C. Situational-contingency theory	_____ ABC model—analysis of clear expectations, behavioral change, and analysis of consequences
D. Hierarchy of needs	_____ Leaders have certain characteristics that inspire

Answers to this chapter begin on page 11.

Column A	Column B
E. Two-factor theory	_____ Leadership depends on the task, the leader's interpersonal skills, and the work to be done
F. Expectancy theory	_____ Leaders have to achieve relationships and understand the work environment
G. Organizational behavior modification	_____ Working conditions are important for motivation of employees

 eResource 1-4: To supplement their understanding of motivation, the class reviews the *Principles of Motivation*: http://goo.gl/PWq8W

Dr. Bennett tells the learners that another common theory in leadership is *complexity theory*. Complexity theory recognizes that many different systems function at once within an organization, and that relationships within those systems are important. For instance, a nurse has relationships with patients and families, managers, pharmacists, lab technicians, dietary staff, and others, and when there is a problem a solution is sought through interaction and innovation. The five principles of complexity theory are:

- Develop networks within and beyond the organization
- Shared governance among workers is preferred over hierarchical decision making
- Find a distinguishing attribute "tag" for the organization and use it to motivate
- Leaders need to find the most positive working networks in the organization to make changes
- Look at the system as a whole with short- and long-term goals and recognize both the measurable and nonmeasurable data

Jacob asks Dr. Bennett to give him an example of complexity theory. Here is the example:

A nurse on a medical-surgical unit has to draw a blood specimen into a heparinized tube on a patient who is a difficult stick. The nurse obtains the blood and labels the tube in the room. On her way to the pneumonic tube, the nurse is called to help with a patient who has fallen. After the fallen patient is placed back in bed, the nurse sends the blood to the laboratory. An hour later the lab calls the unit and asks for a new specimen because the blood is clotted. The nurse states that the lab let the blood sit too long and the lab states that the blood was sent clotted. The nurse manager listens to both sides. Using the five principles of complexity theory, the issue would be dealt with in the following manner.

Answers to this chapter begin on page 11.

Exercise 1-10: *Matching*

Match the complexity theory concept in Column A to the description or solution in Column B.

Column A	Column B
A. Developing networks	_____ The nurse looks for "efficiency" in the blood specimen process
B. Shared governance	_____ The entire organization looks at the developed process to see if it will fit other departments
C. Naming an attribute or "tag"	_____ The nursing manager asks the staff to problem solve since lab issues are recurring
D. Emerge or engage in organization	_____ The nurse meets with the lab technician
E. Address the big picture	_____ The nurse and lab technician try a new system

Dr. Bennett introduces two other theories that are currently used to describe leadership in health care organizations: *chaos* and *quantum* theories. Table 1-1 shows the key elements of both theories.

Table 1-1: Key Points of Chaos and Quantum Theories

	Chaos Theory	Quantum Theory
Organizational level	Organizations are dynamic and unpredictable	Uses science to understand that systems want order but that order is not linear or predicable
Nursing unit level	Growth comes from disequilibrium, not from status quo	Relationships between members are important
Individual nurse level	Challenges are opportunities for success	Individuals need the opportunity to grow

Jacob raises his hand and asks Dr. Bennett what exactly leaders do in the hospital to keep such a complex system moving in the right direction. Dr. Bennett frames his answer in Gardner's (1990) leadership tasks or things that successful leaders do. As a patient care leader, each nurse will participate in these 10 tasks:

- Envisioning goals—Patient outcomes talked about between nurse and patient/family
- Affirming values—Understanding what the patient would prefer and helping the patient make a decision
- Motivating—Helping the patient in a positive manner move toward a goal
- Managing—Planning holistic patient care
- Achieving workable unity—Helping the patient to achieve the highest level of functioning

Answers to this chapter begin on page 11.

- Developing trust—Being honest and on time in patient care interventions
- Explaining—Teaching patients
- Serving as a symbol—Maintaining a professional relationship and upholding nursing's values
- Representing the group—Participating in nursing issues and shared governance on the unit
- Renewing—Taking care of yourself

Exercise 1-11: *Select all that apply*
Leaders continuously develop and in order to do so they need to have which of the following characteristics?

- ❏ Transparency
- ❏ Self-reflection
- ❏ Being consistent
- ❏ Avoid confrontation
- ❏ Like people
- ❏ Team player

Exercise 1-12: *Multiple-choice question*
Senior nursing leaders in an organization should align their vision with:

- A. That of their team
- B. The current health care trend
- C. Personal philosophy
- D. Organization's mission statement

 eResource 1-5: To learn more about alignment, the class reviews *Mission, Vision, Values, Objectives, and Philosophy of an Organization:* http://goo.gl/zvxSF

Beyonce says that she does not know if she ever wants to be a systems leader. She would prefer to stay at the bedside and be a patient leader for a few years. Dr. Bennett says that this is understandable but all nurses are not only leaders of patient care, they also need to be good followers for systems to work effectively. Followership is important and Kelley (1998) has described four types of followers.

Exercise 1-13: *Multiple-choice question*
The follower who is passive and goes along with the leader without questions falls into the category of:

- A. Alienated follower
- B. Sheep
- C. Effective follower
- D. "Yes" follower

Answers to this chapter begin on page 11.

Exercise 1-14: *Multiple-choice question*
The follower who conforms and always supports the leader enthusiastically falls into the category of:

A. Alienated follower

B. Sheep

C. Effective follower

D. "Yes" follower

Exercise 1-15: *Multiple-choice question*
The follower who is passive and hostile but thinks critically about what the leader describes falls into the category of:

A. Alienated follower

B. Sheep

C. Effective follower

D. "Yes" follower

Exercise 1-16: *Multiple-choice question*
The follower who is actively involved and thinks critically about ideas falls into the category of:

A. Alienated follower

B. Sheep

C. Effective follower

D. "Yes" follower

Rosenbach and Potter (1998) also describe follower styles but do it slightly differently. Beyonce laughs when she looks at the titles of followers given by Rosenbach and Potter because she can recognize these types of nurses just from her clinical experiences.

Exercise 1-17: *Matching*
Match the descriptor in Column A with the identifying data in Column B.

Column A	Column B
A. Partner	_____ Good interpersonal skills but neglects his job
B. Contributor	_____ Good relationship with leader and would be able to assume role if needed
C. Politician	_____ Does not usually support leader but does what he is told
D. Subordinate	_____ Does a good job but does not agree with leader

Answers to this chapter begin on page 11.

The class discusses in length about being an effective leader and an effective follower. They ask if a necessary competency is *emotional intelligence*. Emotional intelligence is more than IQ; it takes:

- Knowing one's emotions
- Managing emotions
- Motivating oneself
- Recognizing emotions in others
- Handling relationships

eResource 1-6: Dr. Bennett shows the class a video that provides a brief overview of *Skills for Developing Emotional Intelligence:* http://goo.gl/qAAvS

Exercise 1-18: *Multiple-choice question*

A new nurse is given an assignment that she perceives is difficult. Using emotional intelligence to solve the dilemma would best be demonstrated by:

    A. Telling the charge nurse that she is not doing the assignment and why

    B. Calling the supervisor to report the unsafe patient condition

    C. Asking the other nurses what their assignments are

    D. Asking the charge nurse to discuss the assignment with her

eResource 1-7: To further enhance the students' understanding of emotional intelligence, Dr. Bennett shows the class a video vignette demonstrating emotional intelligence in practice: http://goo.gl/bsIgY

eResource 1-8: The instructor asks the class to take an emotional intelligence test to see what their own emotional intelligence score is: http://goo.gl/8NJ1R

Beyonce and Jacob agree that learning the differences among leaders, managers, and followers was an eye-opening day in class. Next week they are going to learn about organizational systems and get more information about how an actual nursing unit is staffed and how it runs. The method of care delivery never really occurred to them before as students because they were so intent on getting their patient assignments done. Now they understand that for their future careers, this information is important!

Answers to this chapter begin on page 11.

Answers

Exercise 1-1: *Multiple-choice question*
All nurses are leaders in patient health care primarily because they:
A. Have the most education—NO, this is not always true.
B. Administrate hospitals—NO, they do this sometimes but the administrator is not always a nurse.
C. **Know the patient the best—YES, nurses are the ones who tend to understand the patient's needs the best.**
D. Are' with the patients the longest—NO, this is true but not the reason; the reason is that they assess the patient holistically.

Exercise 1-2: *Fill-in*
Place an "L" for leader and an "M" for manager beside the traits listed below.
  L   Change agent
  L   Future oriented
  M   Time oriented
  L   Visionary
  M   Organizes
  M   Budgets
  L   Motivates
  M   Consistency

Exercise 1-3: *Select all that apply*
Select the practices that are attributed to a transformational leader:
☒ **Challenges the status quo—YES, leaders are risk takers.**
☐ Enforces changes—NO, managers do the day-to-day reinforcement.
☐ Rewards employees who meet goals—NO, managers use behavioral modification to promote change, leaders use inspiration.
☒ **Motivates and inspires—YES, leaders motivate by inspiration!**
☒ **Empowers others—YES, leaders help others see their talents.**
☐ Communicates down the organizational channels—NO, this is hierarchical and leaders use direct communication.

Exercise 1-4: *Matching*

Match the term in Column A to the description in Column B.

Column A		Column B
A. Autocratic	__D__	Group makes the decisions, not the leader
B. Democratic	__H__	Focuses on visions and values
C. Great-man theory	__B__	Equally considers group opinion
D. Laissez-faire	__F__	Characteristics that enable the leader
E. Situational leaders	__C__	Born with an ability to lead others
F. Trait leaders	__A__	Leader makes all the decisions
G. Transactional	__G__	Traditional leadership style
H. Transformational	__E__	An event determines the leader

Exercise 1-5: *Multiple-choice question*

A nurse requests a schedule change due to a family issue. The nurse manager states, "Find someone to switch with you." The nurse manager is demonstrating what type of leadership style?

A. Autocratic—NO, the manager is not directing.

B. Democratic—NO, the manager is not sharing responsibility.

C. **Laissez-faire—YES, the manager is not involved.**

D. Transformational—NO, the manager is not being inspirational.

Exercise 1-6: *Multiple-choice question*

A nurse requests a schedule change due to a family issue. The nurse manager states, "You cannot change the schedule without going through the staffing office." The nurse manager is demonstrating what type of leadership style?

A. **Autocratic—YES, the manager is directing.**

B. Democratic—NO, the manager is not sharing responsibility.

C. Laissez-faire—NO, the manager is telling the nurse what to do.

D. Transformational—NO, the manager is not being inspirational.

Exercise 1-7: *Multiple-choice question*

A nurse requests a schedule change due to a family issue. The nurse manager states, "Let's develop a system to be proactive for all the staff when things like this happen." The nurse manager is demonstrating what type of leadership style?

A. Autocratic—NO, the manager is not directing.

B. Democratic—NO, the manager is not sharing responsibility.

C. Laissez-faire—NO, the manager is sharing responsibility.

D. **Transformational—YES, the manager is being inspirational.**

Exercise 1-8: *Multiple-choice question*

A nurse requests a schedule change due to a family issue. The nurse manager states, "If you can't come in, we will figure it out." The nurse manager is demonstrating what type of leadership style?

A. Autocratic—NO, the manager is not telling the nurse what to do.

B. **Democratic—YES, the manager is working with the nurse to solve the issue.**

C. Laissez-faire—NO, the manager is not leaving the nurse to do it alone.

D. Transformational—NO, there are no inspirational ideas as of yet.

Exercise 1-9: *Matching*

Match the theory in Column A with the key points of the theory in Column B.

Column A		Column B
A. Trait theory	**F**	Good outcomes motivate people
B. Style theory	**D**	Physiological needs must be taken care of first
C. Situational-contingency theory	**G**	ABC model—analysis of clear expectations, behavioral change, and analysis of consequences
D. Hierarchy of needs	**A**	Leaders have certain characteristics that inspire
E. Two-factor theory	**C**	Leadership depends on the task, the leader's interpersonal skills, and the work to be done
F. Expectancy theory	**B**	Leaders have to achieve relationships and understand the work environment
G. Organizational behavior modification	**E**	Working conditions are important for motivation of employees

Exercise 1-10: *Matching*

Match the complexity theory concept in Column A to the description or solution in Column B.

Column A		Column B
A. Developing networks	**C**	The nurse looks for "efficiency" in the blood specimen process
B. Shared governance	**E**	The entire organization looks at the developed process to see if it will fit other departments
C. Naming an attribute or "tag"	**B**	The nursing manager asks the staff to problem solve since lab issues are recurring
D. Emerge or engage in organization	**A**	The nurse meets with the lab tech
E. Address the big picture	**D**	The nurse and lab tech try a new system

Exercise 1-11: *Select all that apply*

Leaders continuously develop and in order to do so they need to have which of the following characteristics?

☒ **Transparency—YES, leaders do not keep information away from the team.**

☒ **Self-reflection—YES, this is necessary in order to grow by understanding what things went right in a situation and what things can be improved.**

☐ Being consistent—NO, leaders like innovation and positive change.

☐ Avoid confrontation—NO, leaders are not afraid to confront.

☒ **Like people—YES, leaders should generally be "people oriented."**

☒ **Team player—YES, it is necessary for leaders to be team players.**

Exercise 1-12: *Multiple-choice question*

Senior nursing leaders in an organization should align their vision with:

A. That of their team—NO, the vision comes from the organization.

B. The current health care trend—NO, this contributes to but does not dictate the vision.

C. Personal philosophy—NO, this should align but is not the driving force.

D. **Organization's mission statement—YES, this should be the foundation of the vision.**

Exercise 1-13: *Multiple-choice question*

The follower who is passive and goes along with the leader without questions falls into the category of:

A. Alienated follower—NO, this follower is passive but hostile.

B. **Sheep—YES, this follower is passive and conforms.**

C. Effective follower—NO, this follower is involved and critically thinks.

D. "Yes" follower—NO, this follower goes along but does not critically think.

Exercise 1-14: *Multiple-choice question*

The follower who conforms and always supports the leader enthusiastically falls into the category of:

A. Alienated follower—NO, this follower is passive but hostile.

B. Sheep—NO, this follower is passive and conforms.

C. Effective follower—NO, this follower is involved and critically thinks.

D. **"Yes" follower—YES, this follower goes along but does not critically think.**

Exercise 1-15: *Multiple-choice question*

The follower who is passive and hostile but thinks critically about what the leader describes falls into the category of:

A. **Alienated follower—YES, this follower is passive but hostile.**

B. Sheep—NO, this follower is passive but conforms.

C. Effective follower—NO, this follower is involved and critically thinks.

D. "Yes" follower—NO, this follower goes along but does not critically think.

Exercise 1-16: *Multiple-choice question*

The follower who is actively involved and thinks critically about ideas falls into the category of:

A. Alienated follower—NO, this follower is passive but hostile.

B. Sheep—NO, this follower is passive and conforms.

C. **Effective follower—YES, this follower is involved and critically thinks.**

D. "Yes" follower—NO, this follower goes along but does not critically think.

Exercise 1-17: *Matching*

Match the descriptor in Column A with the identifying data in Column B.

Column A	Column B
A. Partner	__C__ Good interpersonal skills but neglects his job
B. Contributor	__A__ Good relationship with leader and would be able to assume role if needed
C. Politician	__D__ Does not usually support leader but does what he is told
D. Subordinate	__B__ Does a good job but does not agree with leader

Exercise 1-18: *Multiple-choice question*

A new nurse is given an assignment that she perceives is difficult. Using emotional intelligence to solve the dilemma would best be demonstrated by:

A. Telling the charge nurse that she is not doing the assignment and why—NO, this is letting emotions get in the way and causing conflict.

B. Calling the supervisor to report the unsafe patient condition—NO, this is letting emotions get in the way and causing conflict.

C. Asking the other nurses what their assignments are—NO, this is letting emotions get in the way and causing conflict.

D. **Asking the charge nurse to discuss the assignment with her—YES, this is discussing it and using emotional intelligence.**

2

Organizational Structure

Unfolding Case Study #2 ⬛ Roxanne

Dr. Bennett's second class focuses on organizational structures in which new nurses will work. Some of the senior students started their leadership clinical experience this week. One of the learners, Roxanne, was assigned to shadow a charge nurse on a busy medical-surgical unit at the local hospital and to observe the role of the charge nurse. Dr. Bennett starts class and explains the difference between *centralized* and *decentralized* structures in health care organizations. Decentralized structures are used more because they allow *shared governance* at the staff level.

An organizational chart that is flat is decentralized because decision making occurs throughout the ranks; it is sometimes called a *flat structure*. Health care organizations are also divided into *functional structures* with different departments performing different roles such as dietary, laboratory, x-ray, and so on. Product-line structures concentrate on a specific service, such as an outpatient orthopedic surgery center that brings services together under one manager for a specific purpose.

 eResource 2-1: To further clarify these concepts of organizational structures, Dr. Bennett has the class review the Food and Nutrition Organization of the United Nations tutorial, Structure of an Organization: http://goo.gl/YZkQf

Exercise 2-1: *Multiple-choice question*
The nurse understands that when he participates in a unit committee to assist to set up the work schedule, he is working in a system that is:

    A. Centralized

    B. Decentralized

    C. Functional

    D. Product line

Decentralization and shared governance are important for health care organizations to be able to respond to the recommendations of the Institute of Medicine (IOM) report, *To Err Is Human: Building a Safer Health Care System*, which prompted health care organizations to take a good look at how to improve patient safety. Involving the nurses at the bedside through shared governance is one way to get to the root of safety issues.

Exercise 2-2: *Select all that apply*
The IOM has published four landmark reports that have changed health care. Select the four reports:
- ❏ *To Err Is Human*
- ❏ Health Professionals Education
- ❏ The Toyota Model
- ❏ Nursing Education
- ❏ Crossing the Quality Chasm
- ❏ Keeping Patients Safe

Many hospitals have adapted the Toyota Model of organization (Liker, 2004). Toyota uses 14 principles to ensure safety in their product line. The principles cover issues such as transparency, having long-term goals for the company, eliminating waste, and providing every employee the opportunity to stop production if a safety issue is spotted. The model is built on the principles of safety and respect. These principles have been translated successfully into health care organizations.

Outside agencies have affected organizational structure and are part of the current organizational culture of safety. They include the Centers for Medicare & Medicaid (CMS) services that no longer pay for "never events" or patient conditions that are due to poor practice.

Exercise 2-3: *Select all that apply*
Select the 11 "never events" that are no longer reimbursed:
- ❏ Air embolism
- ❏ Blood incompatibility
- ❏ Intravenous infiltrates
- ❏ Catheter-associated urinary tract infection
- ❏ Certain manifestations of poor control of blood sugar levels
- ❏ Deep vein thrombosis or pulmonary embolism after total knee and hip replacements
- ❏ Falls/trauma
- ❏ Wound dehiscence
- ❏ Circumcisions
- ❏ Objects left in during surgery
- ❏ Pressure ulcers
- ❏ Surgical-site infections after certain orthopedic and bariatric surgeries
- ❏ Surgical-site infections after coronary artery bypass graft
- ❏ Vascular catheter–associated infection

Answers to this chapter begin on page 25.

Another agency that has influenced health care culture is the Agency for Healthcare Research and Quality (AHRQ). AHRQ produces research reports for health care workers and consumers, and promotes safety by educating the public.

Exercise 2-4: *Select all that apply*

One of the AHRQ's big consumer safety campaigns concentrated on five steps to safer health care, which include:

- ❑ Ask questions if you have doubts or concerns
- ❑ Switch providers if you do not care for the one you have
- ❑ Keep and bring a list of all medications you take
- ❑ Get the results of any test or procedure
- ❑ Ask for tests or procedures that have not been ordered and are appropriate
- ❑ Ask your provider about which hospital is best for your health care condition
- ❑ Make sure you understand what will happen if you need surgery

The National Quality Forum (NQF) is an organization of providers that has identified 34 safe practices and recognizes nurses as the principal caregivers. The NQF has identified nurse-sensitive conditions that are either patient-centered, nursing interventions, or system-centered.

Exercise 2-5: *Select all that apply*

The NQF patient-centered measures that are nurse sensitive include:

- ❑ Smoking cessation
- ❑ Failure to rescue
- ❑ Pressure ulcers
- ❑ Skill mix
- ❑ Central line–associated bloodstream infections
- ❑ Urinary catheter–associated infections
- ❑ Falls
- ❑ Ventilator-associated pneumonia

The Magnet Recognition Program® of the American Nurses Credentialing Center (ANCC) for hospitals is a special designation granted when the hospital meets certain quality criteria. "The Magnet Recognition Program® recognizes healthcare organizations for quality patient care, nursing excellence and innovations in professional nursing practice. Consumers rely on Magnet designation as the ultimate credential for high quality nursing" (ANCC, 2013, p. 1). The Magnet model is based on the following five components:

- • Transformational leadership
- • Structural empowerment

Answers to this chapter begin on page 25.

- Exemplary professional practice
- New knowledge, innovation, and improvements
- Empirical quality results

Roxanne tells the class that she shadowed a manager in a Magnet-designated hospital and she was surprised that most of the staff was BSN prepared. Dr. Bennett tells Roxanne, Beyonce, Jacob, and the rest of the class that many states are considering legislation called "BSN in 10."

Exercise 2-6: *Multiple-choice question*
Nurses understand that the BSN in 10 legislation will:

    A. Encourage ADN and diploma graduates to go back to school within 10 years

    B. Take licenses away from nurses without their BSN in 10 years

    C. Close associate degree and diploma programs within 10 years

    D. Ensure that LPNs do not work in hospitals in 10 years

Exercise 2-7: *Multiple-choice question*
The BSN in 10 legislation and the recommendation from the IOM that 80% of nurses should have their BSN by 2020 are based on:

    A. Political action taken by BSN schools

    B. Hospitals going for Magnet recognition (AACN, 2013)

    C. Evidence that units with BSN-prepared nurses provide safer care

    D. Community and technical colleges moving to 4-year educational programs

 eResource 2-2: To learn more about quality improvement in health care, the students consult several resources recommended by Dr. Bennett:
- Quality and Safety Education for Nurses (QSEN): http://qsen.org/competencies/pre-licensure-ksas/
- Agency for Research and Healthcare Quality's *Improving Health Care Quality Fact Sheet:* www.ahrq.gov/news/qualfact.htm
- The National State Board of Nurses' response to *The Future of Nursing: Leading Change, Advancing Health* report: http://goo.gl/vquCc
- A detailed overview of Quality Assurance and Management: http://goo.gl/SEJen

Roxanne also tells the group that she was able to observe the charge nurse making patient care assignments for the day. She found that very interesting because the unit uses primary nursing care.

Answers to this chapter begin on page 25.

Exercise 2-8: *Matching*

Match the nursing care delivery strategy in Column A with the descriptor in Column B.

Column A	Column B
A. Functional nursing	_____ One nurse provides care for one patient per shift
B. Total patient care (case method)	_____ A leader is in charge of coordinating a group of licensed and unlicensed personnel to deliver care to a group of patients
C. Primary nursing	_____ Licensed and unlicensed personnel perform specific tasks for a group of patients
D. Team nursing	_____ The nurse is accountable on a 24-hour basis

Dr. Bennett explains to the senior students that it is very important for them to understand the type of patient care delivery system in which they will be functioning so that they can prioritize and delegate appropriately. There are advantages and disadvantages to all four delivery care strategies.

 eResource 2-3: To help the students understand different models of care, Dr. Bennett provides additional resources to help them understand these different models of care:
- CurrentNursing.com's overview of *Models of Nursing Care Delivery*: http://goo.gl/03pOR
- University of North Carolina at Chapel Hill's learning activity *Nursing Care Delivery Systems: Models of Care*: http://goo.gl/SJjOj

Exercise 2-9: *Multiple-choice question*

The nurse tells the associate nurse about the patient's plan of care for the next 12-hour shift along with the expected patient care outcomes. The nurse is working within what type of delivery system?

    A. Total patient care
    B. Primary patient care
    C. Functional care
    D. Team nursing care

Exercise 2-10: *Multiple-choice question*

The nurse is working in a neonatal intensive care unit and is assigned one critical infant for the entire 12-hour shift. This is an example of:

    A. Total patient care
    B. Primary patient care
    C. Functional care
    D. Team nursing care

Answers to this chapter begin on page 25.

Exercise 2-11: *Multiple-choice question*

The nurse has just been given extra patients because a colleague has gone home sick. The nurse has to delegate patients to two LPNs and three unlicensed assistive personnel. The nurse is using what type of delivery strategy?

      A. Total patient care

      B. Primary patient care

      C. Functional care

      D. Team nursing care

eResource 2-4: To support the students' understanding of the nurse's responsibilities in delegation, the five rights of delegation, Dr. Bennett directs the students to review:

      ■ The National Council of State Boards of Nursing's publication *The Five Rights of Delegation:* www.ncsbn.org/fiverights.pdf

      ■ Nursing Currents, *Delegation as a Management Function*: http://goo.gl/RlSsy

Exercise 2-12: *Multiple-choice question*

The nurse is called in to help with a natural disaster and assigns her unlicensed personnel to identify all patients with armbands. This delivery system can best be described as:

      A. Total patient care

      B. Primary patient care

      C. Functional care

      D. Team nursing care

eResource 2-5: To reinforce the importance of delegation and the decision making that goes into effective delegation, Dr. Bennett shows the class a PowerPoint presentation, *Best Ways for the Successful Delegation of Work!* (no audio): http://goo.gl/tztiH

Many variables are taken into consideration to determine the strategy of patient care, including staff mix, patient acuity, and full-time equivalency (FTE) allotment for a unit. An FTE is a position in which a person works for 36 to 40 hours per week. Part-time (PT) positions vary and are expressed in percentages of an FTE, which is calculated at 1.0.

Exercise 2-13: *Calculation*

A nurse who works 3 days a week or 24 hours out of a 40-hour work week would be considered PT at what percent? _____

Per-diem employees are nurses who work as needed for the organization. They are obligated to keep their competency-based education up to date as well as their nursing skills. Many organizations use per-diem nurses when they are short staffed and some have per-diem nurses commit to a specific number of hours per schedule. Schedules are commonly created in 4- or 8-week blocks.

Roxanne also told the class she was able to spend time with the case manager. The nursing case manager is the person who coordinates care for patients in the hospital and beyond. The job can be done by a social worker or nurse depending on the model.

Exercise 2-14: *Multiple-choice question*

Coordination of patient care is important to ensure outcomes and for organizational:

      A. Referrals

      B. Home care visits

      C. Budget considerations

      D. FTEs needed on a unit

Many times case managers use critical pathways or care pathways that contain expected patient outcomes for a specific diagnosis. The pathway of care assists the patient to be discharged on time.

Exercise 2-15: *Multiple-choice question*

A patient with chronic obstructive pulmonary disease develops pneumonia and is kept in the hospital longer than expected. The critical pathway is then said to have a:

      A. Positive variance

      B. Negative variance

      C. Unexpected variance

      D. Additional variance

Roxanne does not have to go back to leadership clinical for 2 weeks, but next week Jacob goes and Roxanne's assignment is to observe and reflect on communication patterns between and among professionals.

Answers to this chapter begin on page 25.

Answers

Exercise 2-1: *Multiple-choice question*

The nurse understands that when he participates in a unit committee to assist to set up the work schedule, he is working in a system that is:

A. Centralized—NO, centralized comes from the main nursing office or the manager.

B. **Decentralized—YES, decentralized originates with the staff.**

C. Functional—NO, this is a system that concentrates on what the organization does.

D. Product line—NO, this is a system that produces a specific product.

Exercise 2-2: *Select all that apply*

The IOM has published four landmark reports that have changed health care. Select the four reports:

☒ *To Err Is Human*—**YES, this was the initial report from 1999 that described that there are 98,000 patient deaths a year in the United States due to hospital errors.**

☒ **Health Professionals Education—YES, this was published in 2004 in order to link education of all health professionals to patient quality care.**

☐ The Toyota Model—NO

☐ Nursing Education—NO

☒ **Crossing the Quality Chasm—YES, this was published in 2001 to improve health care systems to increase patient safety.**

☒ **Keeping Patients Safe—YES, this was published in 2004 and concentrated on improving working conditions for nurses.**

Exercise 2-3: *Select all that apply*

Select the 11 "never events" that are no longer reimbursed:

☒ **Air embolism—YES**

☒ **Blood incompatibility—YES**

☐ Intravenous infiltrates—NO

☒ **Catheter-associated urinary tract infection—YES**

☒ **Certain manifestations of poor control of blood sugar levels—YES**

☒ **Deep vein thrombosis or pulmonary embolism after total knee and hip replacements—YES**

☒ **Falls/trauma—YES**

☐ Wound dehiscence—NO

☐ Circumcisions—NO

☒ **Objects left in during surgery—YES**

☒ **Pressure ulcers—YES**

☒ **Surgical-site infections after certain orthopedic and bariatric surgeries—YES**

☒ **Surgical-site infections after coronary artery bypass graft—YES**

☒ **Vascular catheter–associated infection—YES**

Exercise 2-4: *Select all that apply*
One of the AHRQ's big consumer safety campaigns concentrated on five steps to safer health care, which include:

☒ **Ask questions if you have doubts or concerns—YES**

☐ Switch providers if you do not care for the one you have—NO

☒ **Keep and bring a list of all medications you take—YES**

☒ **Get the results of any test or procedure—YES**

☐ Ask for tests or procedures that have not been ordered and are appropriate—NO

☒ **Ask your provider about which hospital is best for your health care condition—YES**

☒ **Make sure you understand what will happen if you need surgery—YES**

Exercise 2-5: *Select all that apply*
The NQF patient-centered measures that are nurse sensitive include:

☐ Smoking cessation—NO, this is an intervention measure.

☒ **Failure to rescue—YES**

☒ **Pressure ulcers—YES**

☐ Skill mix—NO, this is an organizational measure.

☒ **Central line–associated bloodstream infections—YES**

☒ **Urinary catheter–associated infections—YES**

☒ **Falls—YES**

☒ **Ventilator-associated pneumonia—YES**

Exercise 2-6: *Multiple-choice question*
Nurses understand that the BSN in 10 legislation will:

A. **Encourage ADN and diploma graduates to go back to school within 10 years—YES**

B. Take licenses away from nurses without their BSN in 10 years—NO

C. Close associate degree and diploma programs within 10 years—NO

D. Ensure that LPNs do not work in hospitals in 10 years—NO

Exercise 2-7: *Multiple-choice question*
The BSN in 10 legislation and the recommendation from the IOM that 80% of nurses should have their BSN by 2020 are based on:
  A. Political action taken by BSN schools—NO, this is not the reason, colleges are providing the RN to BSN bridge courses.
  B. Hospitals going for Magnet recognition (AACN, 2013)—NO, this is not the reason, although hospitals with Magnet designation need a certain percent of BSN-prepared nurses.
  C. **Evidence that units with BSN-prepared nurses provide safer care—YES, there is evidence that increasing the number of BSN graduates on a nursing unit benefits patient outcomes.**
  D. Community and technical colleges moving to 4-year educational programs—NO, although some are moving in this direction, this was not the causative factor.

Exercise 2-8: *Matching*
Match the nursing care delivery strategy in Column A with the descriptor in Column B.

Column A	Column B
A. Functional nursing	__B__ One nurse provides care for one patient per shift
B. Total patient care (case method)	__D__ A leader is in charge of coordinating a group of licensed and unlicensed personnel to deliver care to a group of patients
C. Primary nursing	__A__ Licensed and unlicensed personnel perform specific tasks for a group of patients
D. Team nursing	__C__ The nurse is accountable on a 24-hour basis

Exercise 2-9: *Multiple-choice question*
The nurse tells the associate nurse about the patient's plan of care for the next 12-hour shift along with the expected patient care outcomes. The nurse is working within what type of delivery system?
  A. Total patient care—NO, this is when a nurse is only responsible for one shift.
  B. **Primary patient care—YES, this is when a nurse plans out the patient's care for all shifts.**
  C. Functional care—NO, this has to do with dividing up tasks.
  D. Team nursing care—NO, this is a system in which a group of health care providers takes care of a group of patients.

Exercise 2-10: *Multiple-choice question*
The nurse is working in a neonatal intensive care unit and is assigned one critical infant for the entire 12-hour shift. This is an example of:
  A. **Total patient care—YES, this is when a nurse is only responsible for one shift.**
  B. Primary patient care—NO, this is when a nurse plans out the patient's care for all shifts.
  C. Functional care—NO, this has to do with dividing up tasks.
  D. Team nursing care—NO, this is a system in which a group of health care providers takes care of a group of patients.

Exercise 2-11: *Multiple-choice question*
The nurse has just been given extra patients because a colleague has gone home sick. The nurse has to delegate patients to two LPNs and three unlicensed assistive personnel. The nurse is using what type of delivery strategy?
  A. Total patient care—NO, this is when a nurse is only responsible for one shift.
  B. Primary patient care—NO, this is when a nurse plans out the patient's care for all shifts.
  C. Functional care—NO, this has to do with dividing up tasks.
  D. **Team nursing care—YES, this is a system in which a group of health care providers takes care of a group of patients.**

Exercise 2-12: *Multiple-choice question*
The nurse is called in to help with a natural disaster and assigns her unlicensed personnel to identify all patients with armbands. This delivery system can best be described as:
  A. Total patient care—NO, this is when a nurse is only responsible for one shift.
  B. Primary patient care—NO, this is when a nurse plans out the patient's care for all shifts.
  C. **Functional care—YES, this has to do with dividing up tasks.**
  D. Team nursing care—NO, this is a system in which a group of health care providers takes care of a group of patients.

Exercise 2-13: *Calculation*
A nurse who works 3 days a week or 24 hours out of a 40-hour work week would be considered PT at what percent? ____**60% or 0.6**____

Exercise 2-14: *Multiple-choice question*
Coordination of patient care is important to ensure outcomes and for organizational:
  A. Referrals—NO, this is just part of the role.
  B. Home care visits—NO, this is just part of the role.
  C. **Budget considerations—YES, the right coordination of care saves the organization money.**
  D. FTEs needed on a unit—NO, this is not a role.

Exercise 2-15: *Multiple-choice question*

A patient with chronic obstructive pulmonary disease develops pneumonia and is kept in the hospital longer than expected. The critical pathway is then said to have a:

A. Positive variance—NO, this is when a patient outcome allows the patient to be discharged before expected and saves the organization money.

B. **Negative variance—YES, these are conditions that keep the patient longer and use more resources.**

C. Unexpected variance—NO, this term is not used.

D. Additional variance—NO, this term is not used.

3

Communication

Unfolding Case Study #3 ▢ Jacob

The next class topic is communication. The senior students believe this will be a repeat of what they have learned in Fundamentals of Nursing, but in reality the focus of the communication topic is different when one is a senior. Dr. Bennett tells the students that, in leadership, communication is the most important element and that poor communication is the cause for most health care errors. The Institute of Medicine (IOM; 1999) states that health care organizations need to "develop a working culture in which communication flows freely" (p. 180). Free flow of communication is the mechanism to prevent errors.

Jacob's clinical experience this past week was to observe patterns of communication on a busy medical-surgical unit.

Exercise 3-1: *Select all that apply*

The principles of communication include (Sullivan & Decker, 1992):

- ❏ Elaborate on the explanation in different ways so the receiver understands
- ❏ Use simple and exact language
- ❏ Prompt receivers to confirm they understand the message
- ❏ Write the instructions first, then tell
- ❏ Have credibility when sending the message

Jacob tells the group that he witnessed an interaction between the manager and a staff person who is related to a particular lab that was not called to the primary care provider within the appropriate time. He said that he was impressed because the manager spoke to the staff person in private and was an active listener while the staff person explained why the lab wasn't called in.

Exercise 3-2: *Select all that apply*

Active listening includes which of the following activities?

- ❏ Stopping all activity and talking
- ❏ Relaxing yourself

Answers to this chapter begin on page 41.

☑ ❑ Asking for clarification during explanation

❑ Using silence

❑ Reflecting on what is being said

eResource 3-1: To learn more about the communication process, Jacob reads the following on NursingPlanet's website:

▪ *Communication*: http://goo.gl/iQrbj

▪ *Therapeutic Communication in Psychiatric Nursing*: http://goo.gl/UnCdX

During the day Jacob was able to recognize different types of communication styles.

Exercise 3-3: *Multiple-choice question*

The nurse manager states to the staff person, "I am hearing that there were extenuating circumstances at the time the lab values should have been called in" and is demonstrating what type of communication style?

    A. Assertive

    B. Aggressive

    C. Passive

    D. Passive-aggressive

On another occasion Jacob hears a staff member address another staff member in a different manner.

Exercise 3-4: *Multiple-choice question*

A staff member tells another staff member, "I do not know what time I am taking lunch because I am so busy, so you will just have to wait until I get back!"

    A. Assertive

    B. Aggressive

    C. Passive

    D. Passive-aggressive

Exercise 3-5: *Multiple-choice question*

A third staff member heard the previous interaction about taking a lunch break and did not intervene. The third staff member was therefore using what style of communication?

    A. Assertive

    B. Aggressive

    C. Passive

    D. Passive-aggressive

eResource 3-2: To supplement his understanding of the communication process, Jacob watches *How the Communication Process Works*: http://youtu.be/q6u0AVn-NUM

Dr. Bennett also reviews some gender differences in communication between men and women in the workplace that affect the working relationship and interpretation of data. People of both genders report communication challenges.

Answers to this chapter begin on page 41.

Exercise 3-6: *Matching*
Match "M" for male or "F" for female in Column A with the characteristics described in Column B.

Column A	Column B
"M" Male	_____ Being dismissed because of gender
"F" Female	_____ Being subjected to bias if successful
	_____ Experiencing reverse discrimination
	_____ Experiencing difficulty interpreting reactions
	_____ Being excluded from decision making
	_____ Being confused about the ground rules

Dr. Bennett explains to the class that communication is really about relationships and as leaders of patient care, they are going to have to build that relationship with good communication skills in order for their nursing care teams to work effectively.

Exercise 3-7: *Ordering*
As a leader, a nurse will go through four stages of relationship building in order to communicate effectively with team members. Place the stages in order from 1 to 4:

___ Enabling

___ Knowing

___ Directing

___ Meeting

Exercise 3-8: *Fill-in*
When one nursing leader addresses another nursing leader, the mode of communication is considered _____ communication.

e **eResource 3-3:** Dr. Bennet provides the class with a handout that summarizes therapeutic communication techniques that facilitate communication and those that block communication: http://goo.gl/267ZX

Another communication form that Dr. Bennett reviews is email. Emailing professionally and correctly is important and traceable. Email etiquette is extremely important in professional situations in order to protect patients and ensure that Health Insurance Portability and Accountability Act (HIPAA) regulations are not violated.

Exercise 3-9: *Select all that apply*
Select the appropriate rules for email etiquette:

☐ Proofread

☐ Forward the entire email trail

☐ Use lowercase letters

☐ Use emoticons

☐ Reply all to agree to something

☐ Do not send large attachments

Answers to this chapter begin on page 41.

After a class break Dr. Bennett begins to discuss *conflict management*. Conflict management is a necessary skill for nurse leaders to have in order for them to be patient advocates and ensure patient safety. Health care institutions are stressful work environments that can easily trigger conflict because professionals are dealing with important decisions all day long. Negative communication patterns among professionals add to the stress of the environment and set up opportunity for mistakes. Figure 3-1 demonstrates the negative communication cycle.

Figure 3-1:   Negative Communication Style

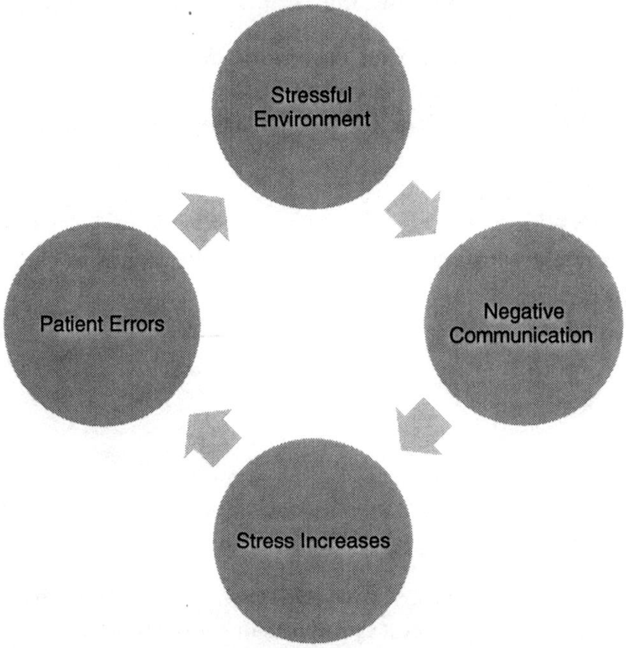

Leaders are guided in conflict management by three principles:

- You cannot change a person's behavior; behavioral patterns are long-standing and may need professional intervention
- You must confront the behavior or it will continue in the work environment
- Leaders can use skills to deal with difficult behavior

eResource 3-4: Dr. Bennett shows the students the American Health Lawyers Association publication *Conflict Management Toolkit*: http://goo.gl/PdghM

Dr. Bennett goes on to describe several types of difficult behavior as witnessed in professionals.

Answers to this chapter begin on page 41.

Exercise 3-10: *Matching*
Match the label in Column A to the description of the behavior in Column B.

Column A	Column B
A. Hostile aggressive	_____ Want to please everyone
B. Complainers or negativism	_____ Cannot choose a course of action
C. Silent and unresponsive	_____ Demeaning and blaming
D. Super-agreeable	_____ Impressed by their own views
E. Know-it-alls	_____ Criticize and are unsatisfied
F. Indecisive	_____ Do not participate

 eResource 3-5: To reinforce the class's understanding of conflict resolution, Dr. Bennett has them pair up and complete a conflict resolution learning activity: http://goo.gl/rv6Ax

Conflicts are more often the result of different personalities, differences in personal needs, continuously unresolved issues, and issues of workload.

Exercise 3-11: *Multiple-choice question*
Nurse A is working with Nurse B. Nurse A overanalyzes situations and checks all the details twice, while Nurse B is action oriented and likes to get things done. Nurses A and B often get into conflicts related to:
- A. Personality differences
- B. Differences in personal needs
- C. Continuously unresolved issues
- D. Issues of workload

Exercise 3-12: *Multiple-choice question*
A conflict arises again between Nurse A and Nurse B over the holiday schedule and who deserves a major holiday off this year. This type of conflict can best be classified as:
- A. Personality differences
- B. Differences in personal needs
- C. Continuously unresolved issues
- D. Issues of workload

Exercise 3-13: *Multiple-choice question*
Nurse B complains to the manager that this is the second day that she has been on first admission assignment. This conflict relates to:
- A. Personality differences
- B. Differences in personal needs
- C. Continuously unresolved issues
- D. Issues of workload

Answers to this chapter begin on page 41.

Exercise 3-14: *Multiple-choice question*

Nurse A needs the Fourth of July off for a picnic she attends every year but it is her turn to work. This conflict can be classified as:

    A. Personality differences

    B. Differences in personal needs

    C. Continuously unresolved issues

    D. Issues of workload

Understanding where conflicts come from is the first step in conflict resolution. The next step is to identify the issues in the conflict and gather information about the issues. A leader also reflects on how the conflict affects her and if she has past experiences with it. There are several ways that people choose to deal with conflict.

Exercise 3-15: *Matching*

Match the word in Column A to the description in Column B.

    A. Avoidance   _____ Takes negotiating skill

    B. Accommodating   _____ Finding shared goals to reinforce

    C. Competing   _____ Postponing the conflict

    D. Compromising   _____ Pursuing own needs in a conflict

    E. Collaborating   _____ Satisfying the other person in the conflict

Dr. Bennett tells the students that the best method he has found for dealing with conflict is to think about it, try to find the "root cause," ask the involved person to meet in a private space, and confront the person in a systematic manner. First, compliment the person on something he or she does well; second, directly tell the person about the conflict; and finish by saying that you are sure it will not happen again or that a solution can be reached. This manner of directly dealing with conflict with another health care professional works by getting issues out in the open without devaluing the person. Lastly, you cannot hold a grudge; you need to move on and leave it in the past as long as the behavior is not repeated.

 eResource 3-6: The class reads a handout provided by Dr. Bennett that provides an overview of conflict resolution skills: http://goo.gl/Ymgui

Beyonce raises her hand and asks what happens if the person does not change or gets annoyed and fights with you. What do you do?

Exercise 3-16: *Multiple-choice question*

Conflict resolution strategies have been ineffective with a nursing colleague. The nurse should therefore:

    A. Avoid the colleague in the future

    B. Ask to be reassigned to another unit

    C. Address the colleague again

    D. Report the interaction to the nurse manager

Jacob raises his hand in class and states that he has trouble sometimes explaining to the patient or the patient's family discharge instructions. Jacob provides the following case that happened to him this past clinical experience. He was participating in discharge instructions with a patient, an 86-year-old man diagnosed with chronic obstructive pulmonary disease (COPD). The patient's younger sister (76 years old) and 81-year-old wife were present. Jacob was explaining to the patient that the capsule goes into the inhaler and is taken that way. The patient thought that he would be able to swallow the pill if he forgot to "do his inhaler in the a.m." Jacob explained that this was a safety issue for an elderly patient, which it surely was! Also, the patient's wife asked Jacob if her husband's breathing will improve and Jacob did not know how to respond to the question. The class discussed multiple issues surrounding these dilemmas, such as poly-pharmacy, HIPAA, and early hospital discharges.

Exercise 3-17: *Multiple-choice question*
The patient with COPD described by Jacob in the class discussion should have a referral for:
>   A. Speech therapist
>   B. Occupational therapy
>   C. Cognitive evaluation
>   D. Home health aide

Exercise 3-18: *Multiple-choice question*
The best response to the COPD patient's wife who asked if her husband's breathing will improve would be:
>   A. "No, COPD is chronic and gets worse as time goes on."
>   B. "Yes, the inhaler will make it better."
>   C. "No, it is a chronic disease but the inhaler should increase the effectiveness of his breathing."
>   D. "Yes, COPD can be managed and new drugs are coming out all the time."

Dr. Bennett agrees that patient communication is a special type of communication that must be addressed carefully in the clinical area. Patients are customers and customer service is important for survival of the institution.

Exercise 3-19: *Multiple-choice question*
A nurse is caring for a 90-year-old patient who speaks Spanish at home but understands a little conversational English. The nurse is providing discharge instructions and should:
>   A. Speak loudly so the patient can understand
>   B. Ask a family member to be present during the teaching session
>   C. Use a Spanish-speaking, unlicensed nursing assistant (UAP) who is familiar with the unit
>   D. Request an interpreter line to use for teaching

Answers to this chapter begin on page 41.

Exercise 3-20: *Select all that apply*

Patient communication should include the following elements:

❑ Provide prompt and tactful assistance when needed

❑ Use proper medical terminology only in descriptions

❑ Recognize cultural issues in interactions

❑ Maintain openness and honesty

❑ Avoid all nonverbal communication

eResource 3-7: Dr. Bennett reminds the students that it is important to pay attention to cultural values when communicating with patients. "Health care providers who consider cultural beliefs, values, and practices are more likely to have positive interactions with their patients. So, let's review the University of Washington Medical Center's *Communication Guide: All Cultures*": http://goo.gl/S3wFJ

Exercise 3-21: *Multiple-choice question*

If a patient becomes agitated during a conversation, the nurse's best initial response is to:

A. Call security

B. Confront the patient and ask the patient to calm down

C. Ask another nurse to witness the interaction

D. Move to a private area

eResource 3-8: Dr. Bennett shows the class a video that presents the value of therapeutic communication from a patient's perspective, *Qualities of a Nurse—Therapeutic Communication for Nurses*: http://youtu.be/Nipj7PwCjTc

After viewing the video, the students have a better understanding of this important aspect of nursing care. Dr. Bennett also brings up the topic of communicating about the patient.

Exercise 3-22: *Ordering*

Place the following communication steps in order from 1 to 6:

___ A for Assessment

___ I for Introduction

___ R for Read back

___ R for Recommendation

___ B for Background

___ S for Situation

Answers to this chapter begin on page 41.

Exercise 3-23: *Multiple-choice question*

Before calling a primary care provider about a patient's condition, the nurse should always:

    A. Assess the patient
    B. Ask the nurse on the previous shift what happened
    C. Call the nursing supervisor
    D. Document the condition

Dr. Bennett discusses how electronic charting has changed the way nurses receive patient orders from primary care providers.

Exercise 3-24: *Multiple-choice question*

The term CPOE in electronic medical records stands for:

    A. Continuous physician order entry
    B. Computerized physician order entry
    C. Computerized provider order entry
    D. Continuous provider organization entry

Jacob tells the class he witnessed a primary nurse taking a verbal order over the phone. He was very impressed with the nurse's procedure for taking the order and said the nurse was a good role model.

Exercise 3-25: *Ordering*

Place the following procedure of taking verbal orders in the correct sequence from 1 to 5:

    ___ Write the order
    ___ Identify yourself on the phone
    ___ Read back the order, spelling out medications and dosages
    ___ Have another nurse listen also if it is a high-risk medication
    ___ Listen to the order

Dr. Bennett also asks the senior nursing class if they have experience reporting a patient's condition to the next shift. Most of the learners have had the opportunity and now call it a "handoff," which is the exchange of essential information about patient conditions. Handoffs are used for other informational purposes.

Exercise 3-26: *Select all that apply*

Nurses use "handoffs" for the following reasons:

    ❑ Shift-to-shift report
    ❑ Transfer of care
    ❑ Family inquiries
    ❑ Change in providers
    ❑ Change in level of care
    ❑ Discharge
    ❑ Grand rounds

Answers to this chapter begin on page 41.

e **eResource 3-9:** To support the students' understanding of the importance of information literacy and its impact on "handoff" and patient safety, Dr. Bennett shows the class a video, *Listen Did You Know?*: http://goo.gl/mhSSl

The learners understand that interprofessional communication can be the difference between life and death for a patient. Dr. Bennett's last PowerPoint slide is a quote from Buddha that he asks the class to reflect on in their professional practice.

"Whatever words we utter should be chosen with care for people will hear them and be influenced by them for good or ill." — *Buddha*

Answers to this chapter begin on page 41.

Answers

Exercise 3-1: *Select all that apply*

The principles of communication include (Sullivan & Decker, 1992):

☐ Elaborate on the explanation in different ways so the receiver understands—NO, say it simply and clearly.

☒ **Use simple and exact language—YES**

☒ **Prompt receivers to confirm if they understand the message—YES, have the receivers verbalize back to you so you are sure they understand.**

☐ Write the instructions first, then tell—NO, explain it to them first.

☒ **Have credibility when sending the message—YES, develop a trusting relationship.**

Exercise 3-2: *Select all that apply*

Active listening includes which of the following activities:

☒ **Stopping all activity and talking—YES, focus on what is being said.**

☒ **Relaxing yourself—YES, this helps you to focus.**

☐ Asking for clarification during explanation—NO, do not interrupt; wait until the end, then ask questions.

☒ **Using silence—YES, this helps comprehension.**

☒ **Reflecting on what is being said—YES, try to find a deeper understanding.**

Exercise 3-3: *Multiple-choice question*

The nurse manager states to the staff person, "I am hearing that there were extenuating circumstances at the time the lab values should have been called in" and is demonstrating what type of communication style:

A. **Assertive—YES, they are addressing the issue without condemning the person.**

B. Aggressive—NO, they are not threatening.

C. Passive—NO, they are confronting the issues.

D. Passive-aggressive—NO, they are not pretending things are fine when they are not.

Exercise 3-4: *Multiple-choice question*

A staff member tells another staff member, "I do not know what time I am taking lunch because I am so busy, so you will just have to wait until I get back!"

A. Assertive—NO, this is aggressive because it is demanding behavior from the other person.

B. Aggressive—YES, this is aggressive because it is demanding behavior from the other person.

C. Passive—NO, this is aggressive because it is demanding behavior from the other person.

D. Passive-aggressive—NO, this is aggressive because it is demanding behavior from the other person.

Exercise 3-5: *Multiple-choice question*

A third staff member heard the previous interaction about taking a lunch break and did not intervene. The third staff member was therefore using what style of communication?

A. Assertive—NO, this is passive-aggressive by ignoring or pretending things are okay.

B. Aggressive—NO, this is passive-aggressive by ignoring or pretending things are okay.

C. Passive—NO, this is passive-aggressive by ignoring or pretending things are okay.

D. Passive-aggressive—YES, this is ignoring or pretending things are okay.

Exercise 3-6: *Matching*

Match "M" for male or "F" for female in Column A with the characteristics described in Column B.

Column A	Column B
"M" Male	**F** Being dismissed because of gender
"F" Female	**F** Being subjected to bias if successful
	M Experiencing reverse discrimination
	M Experiencing difficulty interpreting reactions
	F Being excluded from decision making
	M Being confused about the ground rules

Exercise 3-7: *Ordering*

As a leader, a nurse will go through four stages of relationship building in order to communicate effectively with team members. Place the stages in order from 1 to 4:

__3__ Enabling

__2__ Knowing

__4__ Directing

__1__ Meeting

Exercise 3-8: *Fill-in*

When one nursing leader addresses another nursing leader, the mode of communication is considered **horizontal** communication.

Exercise 3-9: *Select all that apply*

Select the appropriate rules for email etiquette:

☒ **Proofread—YES, always**

☒ **Forward the entire email trail—YES, but only if it pertains to the subject at hand; only one subject per email should be discussed.**

☒ **Use lowercase letters—YES, uppercase is shouting.**

☐ Use emoticons—NO, these can be misinterpreted and are not professional.

☐ Reply all to agree to something—NO, there is no need to clog up other people's email inboxes.

☒ **Do not send large attachments—YES, unless you ask the other person first.**

Exercise 3-10: *Matching*

Match the label in Column A to the description of the behavior in Column B.

Column A	Column B
A. Hostile aggressive	__D__ Want to please everyone
B. Complainers or negativism	__F__ Cannot choose a course of action
C. Silent and unresponsive	__A__ Demeaning and blaming
D. Super-agreeable	__E__ Impressed by their own views
E. Know-it-alls	__B__ Criticize and are unsatisfied
F. Indecisive	__C__ Do not participate

Exercise 3-11: *Multiple-choice question*

Nurse A is working with Nurse B. Nurse A overanalyzes situations and checks all the details twice, while Nurse B is action oriented and likes to get things done. Nurses A and B often get into conflicts related to:

A. **Personality differences—YES, this is a personality difference in style of working.**

B. Differences in personal needs—NO, this has nothing to do with their personal needs.

C. Continuously unresolved issues—NO, this is related to everyday work tasks.

D. Issues of workload—NO, there is no complaint about one having more to do than the other.

Exercise 3-12: *Multiple-choice question*
A conflict arises again between Nurse A and Nurse B over the holiday schedule and who deserves a major holiday off this year. This type of conflict can best be classified as:
  A. Personality differences—NO, this is not a personality or work style issue.
  B. Differences in personal needs—NO, this is not a conflict based on personal needs.
  C. **Continuously unresolved issues—YES, this is related to a continuing issue.**
  D. Issues of workload—NO, there is no complaint about one having more to do than the other.

Exercise 3-13: *Multiple-choice question*
Nurse B complains to the manager that this is the second day that she has been on first admission assignment. This conflict relates to:
  A. Personality differences—NO, this is not a personality or work style issue.
  B. Differences in personal needs—NO, this is not a conflict based on personal needs.
  C. Continuously unresolved issues—NO, this is related to a singular issue.
  D. **Issues of workload—YES, there is a complaint about one having more to do than the other.**

Exercise 3-14: *Multiple-choice question*
Nurse A needs the Fourth of July off for a picnic she attends every year but it is her turn to work. This conflict can be classified as:
  A. Personality differences—NO, this is not a personality or work style issue.
  B. **Differences in personal needs—YES, this is a conflict based on personal needs.**
  C. Continuously unresolved issues—NO, this is related to a singular issue.
  D. Issues of workload—NO, there is no complaint about one having more to do than the other.

Exercise 3-15: *Matching*
Match the word in Column A to the description in Column B.

A. Avoidance   __D__ Takes negotiating skill
B. Accommodating   __E__ Finding shared goals to reinforce
C. Competing   __A__ Postponing the conflict
D. Compromising   __C__ Pursuing own needs in a conflict
E. Collaborating   __B__ Satisfying the other person in the conflict

Exercise 3-23: *Multiple-choice question*
Before calling a primary care provider about a patient's condition, the nurse should always:
  A. **Assess the patient—YES, a good assessment will decrease the need for multiple calls to the primary care provider.**
  B. Ask the nurse on the previous shift what happened—NO, assess the patient yourself.
  C. Call the nursing supervisor—NO, the nurse has the autonomy to make the decision to call.
  D. Document the condition—NO, the nurse needs to do this but not initially.

Exercise 3-24: *Multiple-choice question*
The term CPOE in electronic medical records stands for:
  A. Continuous physician order entry—NO
  B. **Computerized physician order entry—YES**
  C. Computerized provider order entry—NO
  D. Continuous provider organization entry—NO

Exercise 3-25: *Ordering*
Place the following procedure of taking verbal orders in the correct sequence from 1 to 5:
  __4__ Write the order
  __1__ Identify yourself on the phone
  __5__ Read back the order, spelling out medications and dosages
  __3__ Have another nurse listen also if it is a high-risk medication
  __2__ Listen to the order

Exercise 3-26: *Select all that apply*
Nurses use "handoffs" for the following reasons:
  ☒ **Shift-to-shift report—YES, this is used from nurse to nurse.**
  ☒ **Transfer of care—YES, this is used if the patient is transferred.**
  ☐ Family inquiries—NO, this is not appropriate for family.
  ☒ **Change in providers—YES, this is a way to communicate to the new provider.**
  ☒ **Change in level of care—YES, this is an appropriate method to communicate a change in care.**
  ☒ **Discharge—YES, this is an appropriate way to interprofessionally communicate discharge issues.**
  ☐ Grand rounds—NO, grand rounds is a teaching situation that requires extensive background data.

4

Delegation

Unfolding Case Study #4   Beyonce

Beyonce is on her way to experience a leadership clinical day. When she arrives
on the adult medical-surgical unit, she assumes the position of team leader for a
group of patients with her preceptor who is an experienced RN. On Beyonce's
team are an experienced unlicensed assistive personnel (UAP), a recently hired
licensed practical nurse (LPN), and an RN who is experienced in pediatrics and
who transferred to the adult unit 2 months ago. The first thing the preceptor does
is ask Beyonce to review the state's Nurse Practice Act. Practice acts define the
scope of practice for licensed and unlicensed professionals in nursing and can vary
from state to state.

 eResource 4-1: Beyonce also reviews the following:
- Standards of Nursing Practice: http://goo.gl/Rnw2z
- American Nurses Association's (ANA's) Code of Ethics for Nurses with
  Interpretive Statements: http://goo.gl/mSPrD

Next, the preceptor asks Beyonce to define delegation.

Exercise 4-1: *Multiple-choice question*
The best definition of delegation is:
    A. Explaining to a person under your supervision what exactly needs to be
       done
    B. Giving clear directions about what needs to be done to people who report
       back to you
    C. Checking that other people on your team have completed tasks correctly
    D. Providing clear directions about what needs to be done to others but
       checking that it was done correctly

Beyonce then asks the preceptor about accountability in the delegation process.

Exercise 4-2: *Multiple-choice question*

The professional who has the accountability in the delegation process is:

        A. The change nurse

        B. The delegating nurse

        C. The health care provider doing the task

        D. The hospital

Exercise 4-3: *Select all that apply*

The rights of delegation are:

    ❑ Right task

    ❑ Right circumstance

    ❑ Right patient

    ❑ Right time

    ❑ Right direction

    ❑ Right supervision

    ❑ Right person

e   **eResource 4-2:** Beyonce reviews
- National Council of State Boards of Nursing's (NCSBN) publication *The Five Rights of Delegation*: www.ncsbn.org/fiverights.pdf
- The American Nurses Association (ANA) and the NCSBN Joint Statement on Delegation: http://goo.gl/FyVHc

The preceptor goes over the patient care assignment with Beyonce. They have eight patients in their pod or section to whom they are responsible for nursing care for the next 8 hours. The patients are as follows:

1. Room 6A: 48-year-old female, type 2 insulin-dependent diabetic, postop cholecystectomy 1 day who will be discharged
2. Room 6B: 72-year-old male chronic obstructive pulmonary disease (COPD) patient on intravenous antibiotics for bronchitis and pneumonia.
3. Room 6C: 69-year-old female with unstable angina and is on a monitor waiting for a critical care bed
4. Room 6D: 56-year-old male with premature ventricular contractions (PVCs) on a Holter monitor
5. Room 6E: 82-year-old female with congestive heart failure (CHF)
6. Room 6F: 42-year-old female with rectal cancer on chemotherapy
7. Room 6G: 88-year-old male with end-stage renal disease (ESRD) on hemodialysis
8. Room 6H: 26-year-old female with healing burns over 20% of her body who is receiving total parenteral nutrition (TPN)

Answers to this chapter begin on page 59.

Exercise 4-4: *Multiple-choice question*

Which patient should Beyonce assign to the RN on her team?

    A. The patient in Room 6A with type 2 diabetes with an a.m. glucose of 186

    B. The patient with COPD in Room 6B whose arterial blood gases are pH 7.44, PaO_2 86, $PaCO_2$ 35, and HCO_3 22

    C. The patient in Room 6C with a history of angina and indigestion

    D. The patient in Room 6D with PVCs during the night

Exercise 4-5: *Multiple-choice question*

Which patient should Beyonce assign to the LPN on her team?

    A. The patient in Room 6A with type 2 diabetes with an a.m. glucose of 186

    B. The patient in Room 6C with a history of angina and indigestion

    C. The patient in Room 6E with CHF whose potassium level is 3.1 mEq/L

    D. The patient in Room 6F with rectal cancer and a CA-125 level of 190 who is in acute pain

Exercise 4-6: *Fill-in*

Beyonce will not take an assignment but will assist both the RN and LPN with their patient assignment. Select four patients for the RN and four for the LPN from the list below.

_____ Room 6A: 48-year-old female, type 2 insulin-dependent diabetic, postop cholecystectomy 1 day who will be discharged

_____ Room 6B: 72-year-old male COPD patient on intravenous antibiotics for bronchitis and pneumonia

_____ Room 6C: 69-year-old male with unstable angina and is on a monitor waiting for a critical care bed

_____ Room 6D: 56-year-old male with PVCs on a Holter monitor

_____ Room 6E: 82-year-old female with CHF

_____ Room 6F: 42-year-old female with rectal cancer on chemotherapy

_____ Room 6G: 88-year-old male with ESRD on hemodialysis

_____ Room 6H: 26-year-old female with healing burns over 20% of body who is receiving TPN

When the assignments are made for the unit, there are other tasks that come up during the shift that must be delegated to team members in order for the team to be efficient and be able to get to all the patient care needs.

Answers to this chapter begin on page 59.

Exercise 4-7: *Multiple-choice question*

In order to assist with a.m. care, which task should Beyonce delegate to the UAP?

    A. Room 6A: 48-year-old female, type 2, insulin-dependent diabetic postop cholecystectomy 1 day who will be discharged, who needs assistance washing but the family has been complaining for 2 days about the care she is receiving

    B. Room 6B: 72-year-old male patient with COPD on intravenous antibiotics for bronchitis and pneumonia who needs assistance with denture care and setting up breakfast

    C. Room 6C: 69-year-old male with unstable angina and is on a monitor waiting for a critical care bed and needs to be repositioned

    D. Room 6E: 82-year-old female with CHF who wants to go to the courtyard for a cigarette

Exercise 4-8: *Select all that apply*

Which of the following mid-morning activities are *inappropriate* for Beyonce to assign?

    ❑ Have the UAP draw blood on the patient in Room 6F

    ❑ Ask the LPN to change the central-line dressing on the patient in 6F

    ❑ Request the LPN to bathe the patient in 6B

    ❑ Ask the RN to collect a clean-catch urine specimen from the patient in 6H

    ❑ Have the RN teach the discharge instructions to the patient in 6A

    ❑ Ask the LPN to evaluate the breathing of the patient in 6E

Right before lunch, Beyonce's team gets extremely busy. The patient in Room 6C, who was waiting for a critical care bed, codes and Beyonce needs to delegate in order to manage the code.

Exercise 4-9: *Multiple-choice question*

Which task should Beyonce assign to the UAP during the code?

    A. Perform cardiac compressions

    B. Draw a blood gas

    C. Receive orders from the primary care provider who is calling

    D. Transcribe the orders that are now needed

The patient is successfully resuscitated and moved to an intensive care unit (ICU) bed. Another admission is placed in Room 6C. The patient is a 28-year-old female with an open reduction femur fracture who is 6 hours postoperative. Beyonce receives the admission and does the admission assessment while the RN on her team finishes the transfer to ICU.

Answers to this chapter begin on page 59.

Exercise 4-10: *Multiple-choice question*
Which task should Beyonce delegate to the UAP for the patient in Room 6C with an open reduction femur fracture who is 6 hours postoperative?
    A. Transfer the patient to the chair
    B. Turn the patient using the abductor pillow
    C. Monitor the traction apparatus
    D. Monitor the compression boot on the opposite leg

Just when things are settling down and lunch is being brought from dietary, several call bells go off again.

Exercise 4-11: *Multiple-choice question*
Which task would be most appropriate to assign to the LPN?
    A. Give 2 ibuprofen to the patient with COPD in 6B who is uncomfortable from coughing
    B. Clean up the patient (ESRD) in 6G who was incontinent
    C. Help the patient on chemotherapy in 6F into the shower
    D. Check the glucose level on the patient in 6A before she eats lunch

Exercise 4-12: *Multiple-choice question*
What task should be delegated to the UAP?
    A. Give 2 ibuprofen to the patient with COPD in 6B who is uncomfortable from coughing
    B. Clean up the patient (ESRD) in 6G who was incontinent
    C. Change the dressings on the burn patient in 6H
    D. Call the primary care provider for a discharge order for 6A

After lunch the patient in 6A is discharged. Beyonce does the discharge teaching and *medication reconciliation* with her preceptor. The UAP transports the patient and family to the patient discharge area and makes sure the patient gets safely in the car.
    While the UAP is in the discharge area, a new father who is ready to pick up his partner and new infant asks the UAP to help him get the new car seat for their new infant into the car correctly.

Exercise 4-13: *Multiple-choice question*
The best method for the UAP to deal with the task of placing the car seat correctly in the car is:
    A. Assist the new parent
    B. Ask security to assist
    C. Call the nurse on the maternity unit to assist
    D. Ask the parent to read the manufacturer's instructions

Answers to this chapter begin on page 59.

Back up on the unit, the emergency department (ED) calls Beyonce to place another patient in Room 6A. The ED nurse provides a telephone report to Beyonce and her preceptor (Figure 4-1).

Figure 4-1: Telephone Report

I	Hi, this is Tony in the ED. I would like to give your report on a patient that is ready to be transferred to bed 6A. To whom am I speaking?
S	The patient, T. C., is a 24 year-old male who was in a bicycle accident 3 days ago and received a severe laceration of the left forearm, which was sutured in the ED. He was then discharged to home. He has returned with fever and pain in his arm.
B	T. C. is a healthy 24-year-old senior college student. He has no history of hospitalizations or surgery. His family history is significant for late-onset diabetes and hypertension. His nutritional status is within normal limits and his body mass index is 26. He has no known allergies. He is left-hand dominant.
A	His left forearm is swollen, red, and warm to the touch. He is having difficulty bending the fingers on his left hand. His wound is draining scant purulent drainage. There are physician orders in the computerized physician order entry system.
R	The orders are to culture the wound, start an intravenous (IV) infusion of D5½ normal saline solution at 1000 mL every 8 hours, provide pain medication (ibuprofen), and begin gentamicin and clindamycin intravenous piggyback.
R	Beyonce reads back the orders that Tony gave her, with her preceptor listening to make sure she understands.

Exercise 4-14: *Multiple-choice question*
To whom should Beyonce assign the new admission coming to Room 6A with a probable diagnosis of left forearm cellulitis?

    A. Preceptor RN
    B. RN
    C. LPN
    D. UAP

Exercise 4-15: *Multiple-choice question*
Which task should Beyonce delegate to the UAP?

    A. Verify the patient's name and identification before antibiotics are hung
    B. Culture the infected wound
    C. Evaluate the capillary refill in fingers of the left hand
    D. Take the wound culture to the lab

Answers to this chapter begin on page 59.

Exercise 4-16: *Multiple-choice question*
Which assignment would be most appropriate to delegate to the LPN?

      A. Discuss the diagnosis of cellulitis with the patient who is asking questions

      B. Have the patient use his left hand in a therapeutic manner such as writing

      C. Hang the appropriate intravenous piggyback (IVPB) antibiotics

      D. Transcribe newly received telephone orders to the paper chart

After both new patients are settled and initial care has been started on them, Beyonce reviews what tasks her team needs to complete before the end of the shift so they can hand off care to the evening shift (3 p.m. to 11 p.m.).

Exercise 4-17: *Select all that apply*
Of the tasks left to complete, which tasks are appropriate to assign to the UAP?

    ❑ Assist the patient in 6A to wash up since his left hand is not functional and his right hand has an IV

    ❑ Obtain a sputum specimen from the patient in 6B with COPD complications

    ❑ Adjust the weights on the traction that was placed on the patient in 6C

    ❑ Look at the Holter monitor readout for the patient in 6D

    ❑ Revise the plan of care for the patient in 6E with CHF who is progressing well and will possibly be discharged tomorrow

    ❑ Determine if pain medication has been effective for the patient in 6F who is on chemotherapy

    ❑ Ambulate the patient in 6G with ESRD to dialysis

    ❑ Calculate the intake and output (I&O) on the patient in 6H who is on TPN

Exercise 4-18: *Select all that apply*
Of the tasks left to complete, which tasks are appropriate to assign to the LPN?

    ❑ Assist the patient in 6A to wash up since his left hand is not functional and his right hand has an IV

    ❑ Obtain a sputum specimen from the patient in 6B with COPD complications

    ❑ Adjust the weights on the traction that was placed on the patient in 6C

    ❑ Look at the Holter monitor readout for the patient in 6D

    ❑ Revise the plan of care for the patient in 6E with CHF who is progressing well and will possibly be discharged tomorrow

    ❑ Determine if pain medication has been effective for the patient in 6F who is on chemotherapy

    ❑ Ambulate the patient in 6G with ESRD to dialysis

    ❑ Calculate the intake and output (I&O) on the patient in 6H who is on TPN

Answers to this chapter begin on page 59.

At 2 p.m. the patient in 6G with ESRD tells Beyonce that he wishes it were all over and that he cannot stand living like this anymore. Beyonce listens attentively and asks the patient if he has a plan to kill himself. The patient states that he has been collecting pain medication tablets throughout his illness in order to take them all at once at some point in time.

Exercise 4-19: *Multiple-choice question*
The initial action Beyonce should delegate to the UAP for the patient with ESRD in Room 6G is:

    A. Call the primary care provider to give him or her the update on the patient's condition

    B. Ask the psychiatric unit if they have any beds available

    C. Sit with the patient one-to-one on suicide watch

    D. Try to find the patient's stock of medication

Beyonce secures a sitter for the patient in 6G to free up the UAP. The monitor alarm goes off on the patient in 6D who is on a Holter monitor. Beyonce is on the phone receiving orders with her preceptor for the patient in 6G who has suicidal tendencies and cannot get to the alarm. The RN working with her takes care of the alarm and tells Beyonce that it is a functional problem due to the leads falling off.

Exercise 4-20: *Multiple-choice question*
The most appropriate person to ask to place the leads back on the patient in 6D who is being monitored is:

    A. UAP

    B. LPN

    C. RN

    D. Herself

Beyonce and her team are finishing up rounds for their shift and need to complete a few more nursing interventions.

Exercise 4-21: *Multiple-choice question*
Which task should Beyonce *not* delegate to the UAP?

    A. Weigh the patient in 6A who came from the ED with cellulitis

    B. Explain the side effects of gentamicin to the patient in 6A

    C. Take vital signs on the patient in 6D who is being monitored

    D. Document the I&O for the patient in 6A

At the end of the shift, Beyonce reports the major occurrences to the leaders of the next shift. During her report she highlights the major events of the day as the RN and LPN report specifics to the next caregivers.

Answers to this chapter begin on page 59.

Exercise 4-22: *Ordering*
Using the S-A-B-C model (safety–airway–breathing–circulation) and Maslow's hierarchy of needs, place the following reported items in priority order from 1 to 8:

_____ The first patient in 6D coded and was sent to ICU

_____ The new patient in 6A now has traction

_____ The I&O for the patient in 6H was fine

_____ The patient in 6F receiving chemotherapy has had moderate pain control

_____ The patient in 6G is on suicide watch

_____ The patient in 6E with CHF admits to still being a smoker

_____ The patient in 6B is coughing less

_____ The new patient in 6C has a temperature of 102.6°F

When Beyonce returns to class she tells Dr. Bennett and her peers about her day. Dr. Bennett asks her to reflect on the most difficult thing that she had to do in her leadership role and the task that came easiest. Beyonce said that she was surprised at how naturally she could make decisions about which patients should be assigned to whom and reviewing the state Nurse Practice Act was a big help. The most difficult task was telling or asking other people to do tasks. It takes practice to get comfortable in the role in order to communicate effectively to coworkers.

 eResource 4-3: The class reviews the underlying principles of communication by:
■ Taking an Interpersonal Communication Skills Test: http://goo.gl/LbQlC
■ Reviewing *How the Communication Process Works*: http://youtu.be/q6u0AVn-NUM

Exercise 4-23: *Select all that apply*
Effective communication to team members includes:

❏ The task to be done

❏ What the coworker thinks of doing the task

❏ Requesting the follow-up of the results of the task

❏ The time frame in which the task should be done

❏ Directly asking if the task was completed

❏ Telling what the consequences are of not doing the task

Next week it will be Jacob's turn to experience a leadership role in the clinical setting.

Answers to this chapter begin on page 59.

Answers

Exercise 4-1: *Multiple-choice question*

The best definition of delegation is:

A. Explaining to a person under your supervision what exactly needs to be done—NO, this neglects the feedback loop.

B. Giving clear directions about what needs to be done to people who report back to you—NO, this neglects the feedback loop.

C. Checking that other people on your team have completed tasks correctly—NO, this is just follow-up.

D. **Providing clear directions about what needs to be done to others but checking that it was done correctly—YES, this includes providing direction and follow-up.**

Exercise 4-2: *Multiple-choice question*

The professional who has the accountability in the delegation process is:

A. The change nurse—NO, this may not always be the person delegating.

B. **The delegating nurse—YES, the person who delegates the task is accountable for the task.**

C. The health care provider doing the task—NO, he or she is responsible to get the task done but in the end may not be accountable.

D. The hospital—NO, it is the nurse who is delegating.

Exercise 4-3: *Select all that apply*

The rights of delegation are:

☒ **Right task—YES**

☒ **Right circumstance—YES, sometimes called the right situation.**

☐ Right patient—NO, this is from the five medication rights.

☐ Right time—NO, this is not included.

☒ **Right direction—YES**

☒ **Right supervision—YES**

☒ **Right person—YES**

Exercise 4-4: *Multiple-choice question*

Which patient should Beyonce assign to the RN on her team?

A. The patient in Room 6A with type 2 diabetes with an a.m. glucose of 186—NO, this can be handled by the LPN because the person will need subcutaneous insulin.

B. The patient with COPD in Room 6B whose arterial blood gases are pH 7.44, PaO_2 86, $PaCO_2$ 35, and HCO_3 22—NO, these are normal findings for the diagnosis.

C. **The patient in Room 6C with a history of angina and indigestion—YES, the symptoms may indicate worsening cardiac problems.**

D. The patient in Room 6D with PVCs during the night—NO, this is a known diagnosis for this patient and the issue is not currently occurring.

Exercise 4-5: *Multiple-choice question*

Which patient should Beyonce assign to the LPN on her team?

A. **The patient in Room 6A with type 2 diabetes with an a.m. glucose of 186—YES, the LPN can administer insulin from a sliding scale.**

B. The patient in Room 6C with a history of angina and indigestion—NO, this patient is unstable.

C. The patient in Room 6E with CHF whose potassium level is 3.1 mEq/L—NO, this patient is unstable.

D. The patient in Room 6F with rectal cancer and a CA-125 level of 190 who is in acute pain—NO, this patient is unstable.

Exercise 4-6: *Fill-in*

Beyonce will not take an assignment but will assist both the RN and LPN with their patient assignment. Select four patients for the RN and four for the LPN from the list below.

RN Room 6A: 48-year-old female, type 2 diabetic postop cholecystectomy 1 day who will be discharged

LPN Room 6B: 72-year-old male COPD patient on intravenous antibiotics for bronchitis and pneumonia

RN Room 6C: 69-year-old male with unstable angina and is on a monitor waiting for a critical care bed

RN Room 6D: 56-year-old male with PVCs on a Holter monitor

LPN Room 6E: 82-year-old female with CHF

RN Room 6F: 42-year-old female with rectal cancer on chemotherapy

LPN Room 6G: 88-year-old male with ESRD on hemodialysis

RN Room 6H: 26-year-old female with healing burns over 20% of her body who is receiving TPN

Exercise 4-7: *Multiple-choice question*

In order to assist with a.m. care, which task should Beyonce delegate to the UAP?

A. Room 6A: 48-year-old female, type 2 insulin-dependent diabetic postop chole-cystectomy 1 day who will be discharged, who needs assistance washing but the family has been complaining for 2 days about the care she is receiving—NO, the patient's family is the issue here and the leader needs to take care of the patient and/or family complaints.

B. **Room 6B: 72-year-old male patient with COPD on intravenous antibiotics for bronchitis and pneumonia who needs assistance with denture care and setting up breakfast—YES, this is an appropriate assignment for the UAP.**

C. Room 6C: 69-year-old male with unstable angina and is on a monitor waiting for a critical care bed and needs to be repositioned—NO, this patient is unstable and needs frequent assessment.

D. Room 6E: 82-year-old female with CHF who wants to go to the courtyard for a cigarette—NO, there is no smoking allowed in any facility.

Exercise 4-8: *Select all that apply*

Which of the following mid-morning activities are *inappropriate* for Beyonce to assign?

❏ Have the UAP draw blood on the patient in Room 6F—NO, this is appropriate.

☒ **Ask the LPN to change the central-line dressing on the patient in 6F—YES, this should be completed by an RN.**

❏ Request the LPN to bathe the patient in 6B—NO, this is appropriate.

❏ Ask the RN to collect a clean-catch urine specimen from the patient in 6H—NO, this is appropriate.

❏ Have the RN teach the discharge instructions to the patient in 6A—NO, this is appropriate.

☒ **Ask the LPN to evaluate the breathing of the patient in 6E—YES, this is an assessment that should be completed by an RN.**

Exercise 4-9: *Multiple-choice question*

Which task should Beyonce assign to the UAP during the code?

A. **Perform cardiac compressions—YES, UAPs have training in cardiopulmonary resuscitation.**

B. Draw a blood gas—NO, this is a task for an RN.

C. Receive orders from the primary care provider who is calling—NO, this is a task for an RN.

D. Transcribe the orders that are now needed—NO, this is a task for a unit secretary.

Exercise 4-10: *Multiple-choice question*
Which task should Beyonce delegate to the UAP for the patient in Room 6C with an open reduction femur fracture who is 6 hours postoperative?
   A. Transfer the patient to the chair—NO, this is inappropriate for this patient.
   B. **Turn the patient using the abductor pillow—YES, this is appropriate.**
   C. Monitor the traction apparatus—NO, this should be done by the RN.
   D. Monitor the compression boot on the opposite leg—NO, this should be done by the RN.

Exercise 4-11: *Multiple-choice question*
Which task would be most appropriate to assign to the LPN?
   A. Give 2 ibuprofen to the patient with COPD in 6B who is uncomfortable from coughing—**YES, medication administration is within the licensure of an LPN.**
   B. Clean up the patient (ESRD) in 6G who was incontinent—NO, this would be a task better assigned to the UAP.
   C. Help the patient on chemotherapy in 6F into the shower—NO, this would be a task better assigned to the UAP.
   D. Check the glucose level on the patient in 6A before she eats lunch—NO, this would be a task better assigned to the UAP.

Exercise 4-12: *Multiple-choice question*
What task should be delegated to the UAP?
   A. Give 2 ibuprofen to the patient with COPD in 6B who is uncomfortable from coughing—NO, this would be a task better assigned to the LPN because UAPs under normal circumstances do not administer medications. (There are some states that allow UAPs, called "medication technicians," to administer routine medications in long-term care facilities.)
   B. **Clean up the patient (ESRD) in 6G who was incontinent—YES, this is an appropriate task.**
   C. Change the dressings on the burn patient in 6H—NO, dressing changes are usually done by a licensed person because they involve assessment of the wound.
   D. Call the primary care provider for a discharge order for 6A—NO, a UAP cannot take verbal orders.

Exercise 4-13: *Multiple-choice question*
The best method for the UAP to deal with the task of placing the car seat correctly in the car is:
   A. Assist the new parent—NO, this is only done by a car-seat technician, who is a person who has been educated with an official course.
   B. Ask security to assist—NO, this is only done by a car-seat technician.

C. Call the nurse on the maternity unit to assist—NO, this is only done by a car-seat technician.

D. **Ask the parent to read the manufacturer's instructions—YES, the parents are responsible for the task of placing the infant correctly in the car seat.**

Exercise 4-14: *Multiple-choice question*

To whom should Beyonce assign the new admission coming to Room 6A with a probable diagnosis of left forearm cellulitis?

A. Preceptor RN—NO, she is the team leader with Beyonce.

B. RN—NO, the RN has four patients already and there is nothing in the care of the new patient that cannot be completed by an LPN.

C. **LPN—YES, the LPN can hang intravenous antibiotics and obtain cultures.**

D. UAP—NO, this is not in the practice scope of a UAP.

Exercise 4-15: *Multiple-choice question*

Which task should Beyonce delegate to the UAP?

A. Verify the patient's name and identification before antibiotics are hung—NO, this must be done by the nurse administering the medication.

B. Culture the infected wound—NO, this should be done by a licensed professional.

C. Evaluate the capillary refill in fingers of the left hand—NO, this should be done by an RN.

D. **Take the wound culture to the lab—YES, this is an appropriate task.**

Exercise 4-16: *Multiple-choice question*

Which assignment would be most appropriate to delegate to the LPN?

A. Discuss the diagnosis of cellulitis with the patient who is asking questions—NO, this is teaching and should be done by an RN.

B. Have the patient use his left hand in a therapeutic manner such as writing—NO, this is a task for an occupational therapist.

C. **Hang the appropriate intravenous piggyback (IVPB) antibiotics—YES, this is within the role of an LPN.**

D. Transcribe newly received telephone orders to the paper chart—NO, this can be done by a unit secretary.

Exercise 4-17: *Select all that apply*

Of the tasks left to complete, which tasks are appropriate to assign to the UAP?

☒ **Assist the patient in 6A to wash up since his left hand is not functional and his right hand has an IV—YES, this is personal care and can be done by an UAP.**

☒ **Obtain a sputum specimen from the patient in 6B with COPD complications—YES, collecting routine cultures can be done by a UAP.**

☐ Adjust the weights on the traction that was placed on the patient in 6C—NO, this should be done by a licensed professional because of the risk to the patient involved.

❏ Look at the Holter monitor readout for the patient in 6D—NO, this is evaluating a monitor strip.

❏ Revise the plan of care for the patient in 6E with CHF who is progressing well and will possibly be discharged tomorrow—NO, only RNs can plan care.

❏ Determine if pain medication has been effective for the patient in 6F who is on chemotherapy—NO, this is collecting data about the effectiveness of treatment.

☒ **Ambulate the patient in 6G with ESRD to dialysis—YES, this is an appropriate task that the UAP is trained to do.**

☒ **Calculate the intake and output (I&O) on the patient in 6H who is on TPN—YES, this is an appropriate task that the UAP is trained to do.**

Exercise 4-18: *Select all that apply*

Of the tasks left to complete, which tasks are appropriate to assign to the LPN?

❏ Assist the patient in 6A to wash up since his left hand is not functional and his right hand has an IV—NO, this is a task that the UAP is trained to do.

❏ Obtain a sputum specimen from the patient in 6B with COPD complications—NO, this is a task that the UAP is trained to do, collection of routine cultures.

☒ **Adjust the weights on the traction that was placed on the patient in 6C—YES, a licensed person should be responsible for this task.**

❏ Look at the Holter monitor readout for the patient in 6D—NO, an RN should evaluate a monitor strip.

❏ Revise the plan of care for the patient in 6E with CHF who is progressing well and will possibly be discharged tomorrow—NO, RNs plan care.

☒ **Determine if pain medication has been effective for the patient in 6F who is on chemotherapy—YES, this is collecting data about the effectiveness of treatment; if the treatment is ineffective, the RN needs to evaluate the patient.**

❏ Ambulate the patient in 6G with ESRD to dialysis—NO, the UAP can complete this.

❏ Calculate the intake and output (I&O) on the patient in 6H who is on TPN—NO, the UAP can complete this.

Exercise 4-19: *Multiple-choice question*

The initial action Beyonce should delegate to the UAP for the patient with ESRD in Room 6G is:

A. Call the primary care provider to give him or her the update on the patient's condition—NO, this should be completed by the RN.

B. Ask the psychiatric unit if they have any beds available—NO, this is not the priority.

C. **Sit with the patient one-to-one on suicide watch—YES, this is the safety priority.**

D. Try to find the patient's stock of medication—NO, this is not the priority.

Exercise 4-20: *Multiple-choice question*
The most appropriate person to ask to place the leads back on the patient in 6D who is being monitored is:
   A. **UAP—YES, they are trained to do electrocardiograms and monitors.**
   B. LPN—NO, the UAP can do this task.
   C. RN—NO, the UAP can do this task.
   D. Herself—NO, the UAP can do this task.

Exercise 4-21: *Multiple-choice question*
Which task should Beyonce *not* delegate to the UAP?
   A. Weigh the patient in 6A who came from the ED with cellulitis—NO, the UAP can weigh patients and all patients should be weighed on admission.
   B. **Explain the side effects of gentamicin to the patient in 6A—YES, this is teaching and should be done by an RN.**
   C. Take vital signs on the patient in 6D who is being monitored—NO, the UAP can take routine vital signs.
   D. Document the I&O for the patient in 6A—NO, the UAP can do routine vital signs.

Exercise 4-22: *Ordering*
Using the S-A-B-C model (safety–airway–breathing–circulation) and Maslow's hierarchy of needs, place the following reported items in priority order from 1 to 8:
   8 The first patient in 6D coded and was sent to ICU—This patient is already off the unit.
   4 The new patient in 6A now has traction—This is a significant treatment with risk.
   7 The I&O for the patient in 6H was fine—Normal finding
   3 The patient in 6F receiving chemotherapy has had moderate pain control—Pain is a significant nursing concern.
   1 The patient in 6G is on suicide watch—YES, this is first because of safety.
   5 The patient in 6E with CHF admits to still being a smoker—May impact recovery
   6 The patient in 6B is coughing less—Nice to know but not a priority
   2 The new patient in 6C has a temperature of 102.6°F—This is a significant finding.

Exercise 4-23: *Select all that apply*
Effective communication to team members includes:
☒ **The task to be done—YES**
❑ What the coworker thinks of doing the task—NO, this is not part of the decision-making process that needs to be communicated.
☒ **Requesting the follow-up of the results of the task—YES**
☒ **The time frame in which the task should be done—YES**
☒ **Directly asking if the task was completed—YES, this is follow-up.**
❑ Telling what the consequences are of not doing the task—NO, this is not part of the communication process.

5

Evidence-Based Practice

Unfolding Case Study #5 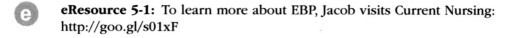 Jacob

Jacob's first clinical leadership experience is following the nurse researcher. The nurse researcher's role is to assist the staff nurses to use evidence-based practice (EBP) to improve patient outcomes.

Exercise 5-1: *Multiple-choice question*
Traditional clinical practice is based in all of the following paradigms except:

- A. History
- B. Research
- C. Pathophysiology
- D. Experience of providers

Exercise 5-2: *Select all that apply*
EBP takes into consideration:

- ☐ Providers' expertise
- ☑ Patient preferences
- ☐ Research findings
- ☑ Best practice
- ☐ Family expectations
- ☑ Cost

> **eResource 5-1:** To learn more about EBP, Jacob visits Current Nursing: http://goo.gl/s01xF

Jacob asks the nurse researcher many questions about implementing EBP. Although he has studied EBP throughout his program, to see it in action is a positive learning experience. The nurse researcher tells him all about the advantages of instituting an EBP program for nurses.

Exercise 5-3: *Select all that apply*

The nursing advantages of implementing EBP in a clinical setting are:

☑ Fewer health care errors

☑ Increased nursing satisfaction

☐ Decreased primary care provider involvement

☑ Establish a research plan for Magnet® recognition

☐ Better communication between patients and nursing staff

☑ Increased patient satisfaction

 eResource 5-2: Jacob remembers a guest lecture the class had last term where the speaker discussed the value of EBP:
- *Evidence-Based Practice in Nursing*: http://goo.gl/0Qh5j
- *Why We Need Evidence-Based Health Care*: http://goo.gl/6rVZT

Jacob's preceptor for the day reviews the levels of evidence with him to make sure he understands the basic components of EBP.

Exercise 5-4: *Ordering*

Order from 1 to 7 the hierarchy of evidence:

__3__ Systematic reviews of correlation/observational studies

__6__ Single descriptive/qualitative/physiologic study

__1__ Systematic review of randomized control trials and nonrandomized trials

__7__ Opinions

__2__ Single randomized or nonrandomized study

__4__ Single correlation/observational study

__5__ Systematic review of descriptive/qualitative/physiologic study

The nurse educator took Jacob up to the first nursing unit and checked her mailbox on the unit. In her mailbox was a form filled out by a staff nurse (Figure 5-1).

Figure 5-1: PICOT Questions Formation

P	Why in the medical-surgical patients of 3 Tower
I	The mechanical blood pressures as opposed to
C	The manual blood pressure readings
O	Seem to be lower
T	When taken one after another?

Exercise 5-5: *Multiple-choice question*

Jacob understands that the "C" in the PICOT questions formation stands for:

A. Correlation

B. Comparison

C. Consequence

D. Complaint

Answers to this chapter begin on page 73.

eResource 5-3: To supplement his understanding, Jacob watches *Framing Your Search: Using PICOT*: http://goo.gl/Lxq8G

The nurse researcher tells Jacob this is perfect timing because there is a hospital research council meeting today. The second nursing care unit they visit is 6th Tower and there is a nursing research program in process that the nurse researcher is overseeing. The project is surveying primary care providers and nurses about their feelings related to using AND (allow natural death) as opposed to DNR (do not resuscitate) when assisting family members of a loved one make end-of-life care decisions.

Exercise 5-6: *Multiple-choice question*
The staff on the unit is discussing the data collection phase of their AND vs. DNR project and are not sure how many surveys they need to collect from health care professionals. This is usually determined by:
   A. The amount of people that work on the unit
   B. The number of patients that are cared for on the unit
   C. A Student *t*-test
   D. A power analysis

 eResource 5-4: For more information, Jacob consults the following:
   ▪ A video, *How to Calculate Samples Size Proportions*: http://goo.gl/cjgc3
   ▪ Russ Lenth's *Power and Sample Size Page*: http://goo.gl/d72G4
   ▪ StatPage.net, *Power, Sample Size and Experimental Design Calculations*: http://statpages.org/#Power

Jacob follows the nurse researcher to an intensive care unit (ICU) that had a recent change of practice for their patient care. A review of the literature demonstrated that using chlorhexidine gluconate baths on patients decreases the transmission of hospital-acquired methicillin-resistant *Staphylococcus aureus* (HA-MRSA). The nursing staff did not feel they had to conduct their own research study because there was ample evidence.

Exercise 5-7: *Multiple-choice question*
Once a practice change is implemented, the next step in EBP is:
   A. Look for the next performance improvement project
   B. Note the number of people that have been affected by the change
   C. Evaluate the process and the data
   D. Organize a review committee that meets once a year

Jacob goes to the research council meeting after lunch with his preceptor. Jacob finds that the council is interdisciplinary. The nursing staff from the 3rd Tower nursing care unit discuss how they will do their project comparison of automated and manual blood pressures on patients.

Answers to this chapter begin on page 73.

Exercise 5-8: *Select all that apply*

The nurse leader understands that EBP is triggered by:

- ☑ Risk management data
- ☑ PI (process improvement)
- ☐ Nurses' curiosity
- ☐ Ideas with low-impact outcomes
- ☑ Identification of a clinical problem
- ☑ Benchmarking data

The research council group discusses how they will collect data for the blood pressure project.

Exercise 5-9: *Ordering*

The nurse researcher guides the nursing staff to use the following steps to complete their project. Place the steps in order from 1 to 6:

- __2__ Find any literature relevant to the issue
- __5__ Evaluate the change
- __1__ Decide if the topic is relevant
- __3__ Decide if there is enough evidence on which to base a change
- __6__ If the change has good outcomes, adopt it into practice
- __4__ Test the change on your specific population

The team decides to take blood pressures every morning both manually and electronically and compare the values. Since blood pressure monitoring is a standard on the unit, it is not a significant change of practice nor is there a significant risk, so they will do it as a quality improvement project. The nurse researcher assists them to make a data collection form and a poster so all staff on the unit are aware of the practice that will take place all next month.

The research council group also talks about survey collection regarding the AND versus DNR terminology, and the staff from 6th Tower are not happy with the amount of surveys being returned. They discuss methods to increase the number of returns.

Exercise 5-10: *Multiple-choice question*

The nurse researcher understands that in order to disseminate the results of a project in a nursing journal, the following criteria must be met:

- A. The results are positive
- B. Participants are each notified of the write-up
- C. Hospital's chief nursing officer (CNO) is aware
- D. Institutional Review Board (IRB) permission for the project was granted

eResource 5-5: To learn more about the protection of human subjects and research ethics, Jacob reviews:

- The American College of Physicians (ACP) *Ethics Manual, Sixth Edition*: [Pathway: http://goo.gl/5qvPt → scroll down and select "Protection of Human Subjects" and review content]
- University of California San Francisco's (UCSF) *Research Ethics* in their publication *Ethics Fast Facts*: http://goo.gl/6A2Je

The group from the ICU reports that the chlorhexidine gluconate baths are going well and after 3 weeks in progress they have not had any new cases of HA-MRSA or any adverse reactions. The practice will continue because the outcomes are favorable.

Another group is interested in finding the best method to raise blood glucose levels on slightly hypoglycemic patients. They state that on their unit, different people do different things such as 4 ounces of orange juice, graham crackers, milk, or orange juice with a packet of sugar mixed in. The group has not had much luck finding any evidence in the literature that supports either practice or any other intervention.

Exercise 5-11: *Multiple-choice question*

The only literature that was found about oral treatment with food for slight hypoglycemia was in nursing textbooks. This level of evidence would be considered:

    A. Level 2—single nonrandomized

    B. Level 5—systematic review of descriptive studies

    C. Level 6—single study

    D. Level 7—opinion of authority

The group proposes an EBP project to produce evidence about the best method of increasing blood glucose by approximately 15 mg/dL. Jacob is interested in how they go about starting a project.

Exercise 5-12: *Multiple-choice question*

The nurse researcher informs them that the first thing the group must do to start the project is to:

    A. Write a project proposal

    B. Ask the CNO

    C. Check with the doctors who put patients on the unit

    D. Hire a statistician

Jacob has a much better idea of how EBP works at the point of care. At the end of the clinical day, Jacob thanks his preceptor and prepares to write up the experience to share with the class the next time they meet.

Answers to this chapter begin on page 73.

Answers

Exercise 5-1: *Multiple-choice question*
Traditional clinical practice is based in all of the following paradigms except:
  A. History—NO, this is basically tradition.
  B. **Research—YES, this is what it should be based on.**
  C. Pathophysiology—NO, this is what historically it has been based on.
  D. Experience of providers—NO, this too is tradition.

Exercise 5-2: *Select all that apply*
EBP takes into consideration:

❑ Providers' expertise—NO, this should not be considered.

☒ **Patient preferences—YES, patient preferences should always be taken into consideration.**

☒ **Research findings—YES**

☒ **Best practice—YES**

❑ Family expectations—NO, this is not a primary driving factor for EBP.

☒ **Cost—YES, the cost of health care is a factor that needs to be considered.**

Exercise 5-3: *Select all that apply*
The nursing advantages of implementing EBP in a clinical setting are:

☒ **Fewer health care errors—YES**

☒ **Increased nursing satisfaction—YES**

❑ Decreased primary care provider involvement—NO, EBP should not decrease any professional's involvement in patient care.

☒ **Establish a research plan for Magnet® recognition—YES**

❑ Better communication between patients and nursing staff—NO, EBP itself doesn't increase communication.

☒ **Increased patient satisfaction—YES, it should increase patient satisfaction since they are part of the EBP process.**

Exercise 5-4: *Ordering*

Order from 1 to 7 the hierarchy of evidence:

__3__ Systematic reviews of correlation/observational studies

__6__ Single descriptive/qualitative/physiologic study

__1__ Systematic review of randomized control trials and nonrandomized trials

__7__ Opinions

__2__ Single randomized or nonrandomized study

__4__ Single correlation/observational study

__5__ Systematic review of descriptive/qualitative/physiologic study

Exercise 5-5: *Multiple-choice question*

Jacob understands that the "C" in the PICOT questions formation stands for:

   A. Correlation—NO, this is a type of statistical analysis.

   B. **Comparison—YES, it is comparing one intervention to another.**

   C. Consequence—NO, this is outcome based.

   D. Complaint—NO, this is how issues may arise.

Exercise 5-6: *Multiple-choice question*

The staff on the unit is discussing the data collection phase of their AND vs. DNR project and are not sure how many surveys they need to collect from health care professionals. This is usually determined by:

   A. The amount of people that work on the unit—NO, this may be a factor but should not determine the data collection process.

   B. The number of patients that are cared for on the unit—NO, this should not determine the data collection process.

   C. A Student *t*-test—NO, this is used to compare means of two groups.

   D. **A power analysis—YES, this is done a priori to determine how many participants are needed.**

Exercise 5-7: *Multiple-choice question*

Once a practice change is implemented, the next step in EBP is:

   A. Look for the next performance improvement project—NO, the current process is still not complete.

   B. Note the number of people that have been affected by the change—NO, this is the outcome process.

   C. **Evaluate the process and the data—YES, the team must see if the change has produced positive outcomes with minimal harm and cost.**

   D. Organize a review committee that meets once a year—NO, this is not part of the process.

Exercise 5-8: *Select all that apply*

The nurse leader understands that EBP is triggered by:

☒ **Risk management data—YES, reducing risk management issues is a must for the hospital.**

☒ **PI (process improvement)—YES, improving performance is a good reason to use evidence to support best practice.**

❑ Nurses' curiosity—NO, this in itself is not a driving force but can lead to a significant PICOT question.

❑ Ideas with low impact outcomes—NO, if it is a "so what" idea there is no need to pursue it.

☒ **Identification of a clinical problem—YES, this is one of the most common reasons.**

☒ **Benchmarking data—YES, it helps to bring data up to benchmarks.**

Exercise 5-9: *Ordering*

The nurse researcher guides the nursing staff to use the following steps to complete their project. Place the steps in order from 1 to 6:

__2__ Find any literature relevant to the issue

__5__ Evaluate the change

__1__ Decide if the topic is relevant

__3__ Decide if there is enough evidence on which to base a change

__6__ If the change has good outcomes, adopt it into practice

__4__ Test the change on your specific population

Exercise 5-10: *Multiple-choice question*

The nurse researcher understands that in order to disseminate the results of a project in a nursing journal, the following criteria must be met:

A. The results are positive—NO, even negative results are valuable to the professional community.

B. Participants are each notified of the write-up—NO, this is usually only done for case studies in qualitative research.

C. Hospital's chief nursing officer (CNO) is aware—NO, although this may be a hospital protocol, it is not a necessary step in all organizations.

D. **IRB permission for the project was granted—YES, it involves human subjects and is invasive.**

Exercise 5-11: *Multiple-choice question*

The only literature that was found about oral treatment with food for slight hypoglycemia was in nursing textbooks. This level of evidence would be considered:

A. Level 2—single nonrandomized—NO

B. Level 5—systematic review of descriptive studies—NO

C. Level 6—single study—NO

D. **Level 7—opinion of authority—YES, this is usually a traditional opinion.**

Exercise 5-12: *Multiple-choice question*

The nurse researcher informs them that the first thing the group must do to start the project is to:

  A. **Write a project proposal—YES, this tells the IRB and the research community what the intentions are.**

  B. Ask the CNO—NO, this may be a consideration but is often not a necessary step.

  C. Check with the doctors who put patients on the unit—NO, this may be a consideration but is often not a necessary step.

  D. Hire a statistician—NO, this can be done later if needed.

6

Triaging

Unfolding Case Study #6 ▪ Roxanne

Beyonce and Jacob describe to the learners in their class their experiences in leadership clinical. Roxanne is scheduled to be the leader for clinical tomorrow, although all the other learners in the class are also participating, as well as faculty and community volunteers. Tomorrow is a regional natural disaster drill. The drill is taking place in the parking lot of the community's baseball field. Today in class Mr. Bennett is reviewing some initial information about disasters that can occur inside or outside the walls of any health care organization. He will also review information the learners will need to participate in the drill.

Exercise 6-1: *Select all that apply*
All health care organizations that are accredited must be able to document that they have a safe environment. The accrediting agencies that enforce these standards include:

- ❏ The Joint Commission (TJC)
- ❏ Occupational Safety and Health Administration (OSHA)
- ❏ Health Resources and Services Administration (HRSA)
- ❏ Centers for Disease Control and Prevention (CDC)
- ❏ Health Insurance Portability and Accountability Act (HIPAA)
- ❏ State Board of Nursing

Exercise 6-2: *Multiple-choice question*
TJC standard of environment of care includes all of the following criteria except:

- A. Management of security risks
- B. Educating staff about hazards
- C. Management of hazardous materials
- D. Educating patients and families about hazards

ⓔ **eResource 6-1:** For more information about TJC, Beyonce has Jacob visit the TJC's website: www.jointcommission.org

Exercise 6-3: *Matching*
Match the agency in Column A with its major purpose in Column B.

Column A	Column B
A. OSHA	_____ Infectious waste
B. Nuclear Regulatory Commission (NRC)	_____ National patient safety goals
C. CDC	_____ Radioactive waste
D. National Institute for Occupational Safety and Health (NIOSH)	_____ Workplace safety
E. Environmental Protection Agency (EPA)	_____ Bloodborne pathogens and workplace safety
F. TJC	_____ Workplace safety

Exercise 6-4: *Select all that apply*
The following materials are considered hazardous waste materials in a health care organization:

- ❑ Intravenous tubing
- ❑ Oxygen
- ❑ Cleaning fluids
- ❑ Chemotherapeutic drugs
- ❑ Total parenteral nutrition
- ❑ Surgical waste

Dr. Bennett provides a case scenario for the class. A hospital worker is splashed in the face with a cleaning agent. The supervisor instructs the worker to rinse off the chemical agent thoroughly and then investigates any other action that should be taken.

Exercise 6-5: *Multiple-choice question*
Investigation of chemical properties and care in emergency situations is provided by:

- A. Departmental supervisors
- B. Bottle label
- C. Material Safety Data Sheet (MSDS)
- D. Product Information Sheet (PIS)

Exercise 6-6: *Multiple-choice question*
One goal of providing a safe environment is:

- A. Decrease worker compensation claims
- B. Preserve the organization's reputation
- C. Maintain employee satisfaction
- D. Document all occurrences

Answers to this chapter begin on page 85.

Dr. Bennett explains the different categories of all-hazard disasters.

- Biological—Natural outbreak of a pathogen
- Chemical—Exposure to a toxin
- Conventional—Bombings or weapons
- Radiological/nuclear—Results of a facility accident
- Cyber—Closes off information systems
- Agricultural—Animal or plant disease

 eResource 6-2: To help the students learn more about steps to be taken after workplace exposure, Dr. Bennett reviews OSHA's web-based training resources, Hazard Communication, with the class: http://goo.gl/bCzTt

Although they have been in-serviced yearly since they have started their nursing education, Dr. Bennett also reviews fire safety with the class.

Exercise 6-7: *Multiple-choice question*
The third step in fire safety protocol is:
- A. Contain
- B. Extinguish
- C. Rescue
- D. Alarm

 eResource 6-3: Dr. Bennett shares with the class a variety of additional web-based resources that provide guidelines for protection of workers and the workplace environment:
- OSHA's Web Library: www.osha.gov/dte/library
- Oklahoma State University's free online environmental health and safety training: http://goo.gl/GFaY0

Another threat to health care workers is security. All organizations have emergency codes that are broadcasted so that all workers are aware of the situation.

Exercise 6-8: *Multiple-choice question*
All organizations use different codes for different incidences because:
- A. It has been the tradition in that place, and changing would confuse workers
- B. There is a lack of regional and state coordination of code names
- C. The codes are specific to each organization purposefully in order that lay-people do not know them
- D. Different accrediting agencies mandate different code names

Dr. Bennett provides the learners with five practice questions about maintaining a safe environment. After they finish their practice test (Figure 6-1) they can check each other's work for understanding.

Answers to this chapter begin on page 85.

Figure 6-1: Organizational Safety Quiz

Name: _____ **Date:** _____

1. A nurse accidentally gets stuck with a used syringe needle; he flushes the skin with water. What is the next action for safety?
   A. Write an incident report
   B. Get permission from the patient to have blood drawn
   C. Notify the charge nurse
   D. Bleed the wound

2. A parent comes to the emergency department (ED) with a toddler because the toddler drank cleaning fluid that was under the sink. What information should the nurse ask initially?
   A. Who was watching the toddler?
   B. Did you call Poison Control?
   C. When did the toddler drink the fluid?
   D. Do you have the cleaning fluid with you?

3. A parent comes to the nursery to pick up her newborn infant. The nursery nurse states, "Your husband picked the infant up 10 minutes ago." The mother states, "I have not seen my husband today." The next action the nurse should take is:
   A. Notify security
   B. Check in the patient's room for the infant and father
   C. Call a code Adam
   D. Describe the person who picked up the infant to the mother

4. An accident victim is brought to the ED and his friends show up intoxicated. The friends are loud and causing a commotion in the ED. The nurse should:
   A. Escort them outside
   B. Call security
   C. Call the local police
   D. Tell them to leave

5. A patient who has been waiting in the ED to be seen brings a handbag up to the nurses' desk and says this was left in the waiting room but she did not see who left it. The nurse should initially:
   A. Get the name of the patient who brought the handbag to the desk
   B. Empty the contents on the desk to visualize
   C. Open the handbag and look inside with another employee
   D. Call security to come

Answers to this chapter begin on page 85.

The learners understand the information fairly well but discuss that in these emergency situations they will be unsure of themselves. Dr. Bennett reassures them that by reviewing the safety principles, they will know what to do in an emergency situation.

Exercise 6-9: *Multiple-choice question*
Which is not a standard level of disaster management?

     A. Preparedness
     B. Recovery
     C. Response
     D. Relief

He then gives them their roles for the following day.

The following day the learners, faculty, and volunteers meet in the parking lot of the community baseball field as instructed. There are ambulances and paramedics, as well as fire and police officers. In a real situation, the Federal Emergency Management Agency (FEMA) would also respond. Dr. Bennett is one of the leaders of the simulation exercise and reads the following situation to the participants (Figure 6-2):

Figure 6-2:   Simulation Exercise

I	I am the emergency team coordinator and will be the person all teams report to.
S	At 7:55 p.m. this evening a bomb went off at the local ball field during a well-attended game. It was ignited in one of the concession stands that is located behind the stands at home plate.
B	The identity or cause of the attack has not yet been identified. There are approximately 300 spectators at the ball game.
A	There are multiple injuries of fans, some life threatening. The fans that sustained the worst injuries were in section B behind home plate. Section A fans down the first base line were injured if they were in close approximation of section B as were the fans in section C down the third base line.
R	Nurses will "tag" victims. Paramedics and primary care providers will begin administering treatment to victims in priority order. Volunteers will assist by escorting unhurt or minimally hurt patients to a shelter off the baseball campus set up at a local church.
R	Participants repeat the orders back to Dr. Bennett.

Volunteers and students are used as standardized patients and there are also manikins simulating injuries. Volunteer workers and paramedics are pulling people (and manikins) from the stands to the open area of the parking lot to be assessed.

Answers to this chapter begin on page 85.

Roxanne is a team leader and has to triage the patients brought to her area so the team can act accordingly. Roxanne uses the tags provided by FEMA to identify and triage patients (Figure 6-3). Roxanne initially has four patients to tag.

Figure 6-3: Triage Tag

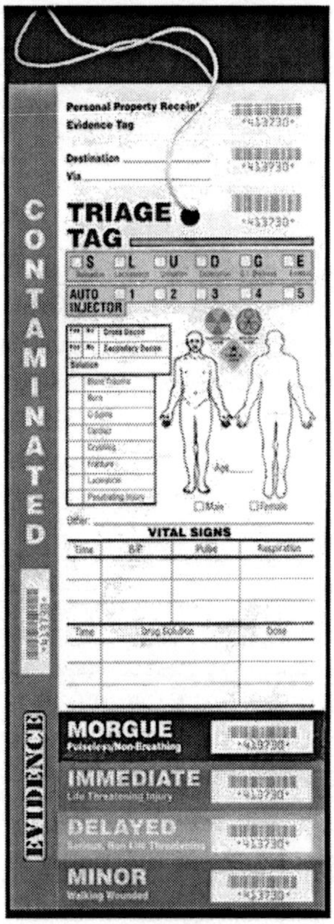

Exercise 6-10: *Matching*

Match the designation in Column A with the patient condition in Column B.

Column A	Column B
A. Morgue (Black)	_____ Closed left arm fracture
B. Immediate (Red)	_____ Superficial laceration of forehead
C. Delayed (Yellow)	_____ Crushing skull injury
D. Minor (Green)	_____ Obstructed airway from embedded debris

The patient with the minor injury is led away to the shelter by Jacob, and Beyonce is assisting the paramedics with the immediate patient. Roxanne is brought another patient by the volunteers.

Answers to this chapter begin on page 85.

Exercise 6-11: *Multiple-choice question*

A hysterical young girl who is bleeding from a large leg laceration is brought to Roxanne. The girl is screaming for her mother who was with her at the game but the mother has not been recovered yet. The best option for Roxanne at this time is to:

      A. Let the young girl run back to the rubble to find her mother

      B. Restrain the young girl so she does not run back in and sustain further injuries

      C. Tag her green and have someone force her to the shelter

      D. Tag her yellow and have someone sit with her one-to-one

Another eight patients are placed in Roxanne's section.

Exercise 6-12: *Matching*

Match the designation in Column A with the patient condition in Column B; designations can be used more than once.

Column A	Column B
A. Morgue (Black)	_____ Compound open femur fracture
B. Immediate (Red)	_____ Burns over 20% of body from explosion
C. Delayed (Yellow)	_____ Back injury, cannot feel legs
D. Minor (Green)	_____ Debris in left eye
	_____ Finger amputated
	_____ Blunt trauma to abdomen, vomiting
	_____ Crushed chest with perforated lungs
	_____ Stroke

eResource 6-4: Roxanne recalls the guidelines reviewed in class the day before the simulation: http://goo.gl/8jbP9

The simulation scenario takes all morning. The activities are engaging and the time passes quickly.

eResource 6-5: To help with their triage decisions in the field, the students have downloaded the CDC's Field Triage Guide for use:
- Mobile App: www.cdc.gov/fieldtriage/mobile.html
- Pocket Guide: http://goo.gl/znwP1

The learners are exhausted by lunch time. Dr. Bennett tells them to get lunch and to come back for debriefing. Debriefing is important after any simulation but especially after a trauma scene. The learners discuss how they feel especially when placing "Black" tags on people. It is very difficult in a society that is focused on

Answers to this chapter begin on page 85.

cure not to try to save someone. The learners also say that they had to use their core nursing principles to get through the experience, which they recount:

- S-A-B-C (safety, airway, breathing, circulation)
- Life before limb
- Physiological before psychological
- Maslow's hierarchy of needs
- The nursing process—assess first!

Answers to this chapter begin on page 85.

Answers

Exercise 6-1: *Select all that apply*

All health care organizations that are accredited must be able to document that they have a safe environment. The accrediting agencies that enforce these standards include:

☒ **The Joint Commission (TJC)—YES, this is an accrediting agency.**

☒ **Occupational Safety and Health Administration (OSHA)—YES, inspects for material safety.**

☐ Health Resource and Service Administration (HRSA)—NO, this is a funding program.

☒ **Centers for Disease Control and Prevention (CDC)—YES, checks for disease outbreaks.**

☒ **Health Insurance Portability and Accountability Act (HIPAA)—YES, regulates the flow of patient information.**

☐ State Board of Nursing—NO, licensing board for professionals, not organizations.

Exercise 6-2: *Multiple-choice question*

TJC standard of environment of care includes all of the following criteria except:

  A. Management of security risks—NO, this is managed.

  B. Educating staff about hazards—NO, this is done.

  C. Management of hazardous materials—NO, this is done.

  D. **Educating patients and families about hazards—YES, this is not a goal.**

Exercise 6-3: *Matching*

Match the agency in Column A with its major purpose in Column B.

Column A		Column B
A. OSHA	**C**	Infectious waste
B. Nuclear Regulatory Commission (NRC)	**F**	National patient safety goals
C. CDC	**B**	Radioactive waste
D. National Institute for Occupational Safety and Health (NIOSH)	**E or F**	Workplace safety
E. Environmental Protection Agency (EPA)	**A**	Bloodborne pathogens and workplace safety
F. TJC	**E or F**	Workplace safety

Exercise 6-4: *Select all that apply*
The following materials are considered hazardous waste materials in a health care organization:

☐ Intravenous tubing—NO

☒ **Oxygen—YES**

☒ **Cleaning fluids—YES**

☒ **Chemotherapeutic drugs—YES**

☐ Total parenteral nutrition—NO

☒ **Surgical waste—YES**

Exercise 6-5: *Multiple-choice question*
Investigation of chemical properties and care in emergency situations is provided by:
  A. Departmental supervisors—NO, they are notified but not responsible.
  B. Bottle label—NO, this does not contain all the information needed.
  C. **Material Safety Data Sheet (MSDS)—YES, this is the mechanism used to know the correct care.**
  D. Product Information Sheet (PIS)—NO

Exercise 6-6: *Multiple-choice question*
One goal of providing a safe environment is:
  A. **Decrease worker compensation claims—YES, this is a large organizational cost that inevitably will raise health care costs.**
  B. Preserve the organization's reputation—NO, this is not a reason.
  C. Maintain employee satisfaction—NO, this is not a reason.
  D. Document all occurrences—NO, this is not a reason.

Exercise 6-7: *Multiple-choice question*
The third step in fire safety protocol is:
  A. **Contain—YES**
  B. Extinguish—NO, this is fourth.
  C. Rescue—NO, this is second.
  D. Alarm—NO, this is first.

Exercise 6-8: *Multiple-choice question*
All organizations use different codes for different incidences because:
  A. It has been the tradition in that place, and changing would confuse workers—NO, this is not the reason.
  B. There is lack of regional and state coordination of code names—NO, this is not the reason.
  C. **The codes are specific to each organization purposefully in order that lay-people do not know them—YES, this is to minimize panic in an emergency.**
  D. Different accrediting agencies mandate different code names—NO, this is not the reason.

Figure 6-4: Organizational Safety Quiz Answers

Name: _____ Date: _____

1. A nurse accidentally gets stuck with a used syringe needle; he flushes the skin with water. What is the next action for safety?
   A. Write an incident report—NO, this is not the next step.
   B. Get permission from the patient to have blood drawn—NO, this is not the next step.
   C. Notify the charge nurse—NO, this is not the next step.
   D. **Bleed the wound—YES, this is the next step.**

2. A parent comes to the emergency department (ED) with a toddler because the toddler drank cleaning fluid that was under the sink. What information should the nurse ask initially?
   A. Who was watching the toddler?—NO, this is not important and will break down the communication.
   B. Did you call Poison Control?—NO, this is important but not the priority.
   C. When did the toddler drink the fluid?—NO, this is important but not the priority.
   D. **Do you have the cleaning fluid with you?—YES, this will help identify the treatment.**

3. A parent comes to the nursery to pick up her newborn infant. The nursery nurse states, "Your husband picked the infant up 10 minutes ago." The mother states, "I have not seen my husband today." The next action the nurse should take is:
   A. Notify security—NO, this is not the priority.
   B. Check in the patient's room for the infant and father—NO, this is a waste of time.
   C. **Call a code Adam—YES, activate the system first!**
   D. Describe the person who picked up the infant to the mother—NO, this is a waste of time.

4. An accident victim is brought to the ED and his friends show up intoxicated. The friends are loud and causing a commotion in the ED. The nurse should:
   A. Escort them outside—NO, this is not your responsibility.
   B. **Call security—YES**
   C. Call the local police—NO, security can do this.
   D. Tell them to leave—NO, confronting a chemically impaired person is not a good idea.

5. A patient who has been waiting in the ED to be seen brings a handbag up to the nurses' desk and says this was left in the waiting room but she did not see who left it. The nurse should initially:
   A. Get the name of the patient who brought the handbag to the desk—NO, this is not a priority.
   B. Empty the contents on the desk to visualize—NO, do not disrupt everything.
   C. **Open the handbag and look inside with another employee—YES, this verifies what you have seen and checks out a potentially dangerous situation immediately.**
   D. Call security to come—NO, this is important but if you wait for security, you waste time.

Exercise 6-9: *Multiple-choice question*

Which is not a standard level of disaster management?

A. Preparedness—NO, this is level 1.

B. Recovery—NO, this is level 3.

C. Response—NO, this is level 2.

D. **Relief—YES, this is not a level.**

Exercise 6-10: *Matching*

Match the designation in Column A with the patient condition in Column B.

Column A		Column B
A. Morgue (Black)	**C**	Closed left arm fracture
B. Immediate (Red)	**D**	Superficial laceration of forehead
C. Delayed (Yellow)	**A**	Crushing skull injury
D. Minor (Green)	**B**	Obstructed airway from embedded debris

Exercise 6-11: *Multiple-choice question*

A hysterical young girl who is bleeding from a large leg laceration is brought to Roxanne. The girl is screaming for her mother who was with her at the game but the mother has not been recovered yet. The best option for Roxanne at this time is to:

A. Let the young girl run back to the rubble to find her mother—NO, this is not safe.

B. Restrain the young girl so she does not run back in and sustain further injuries—NO, restraining is the last resort.

C. Tag her green and have someone force her to the shelter—NO, do not pull her away from the site until her mother is recovered.

D. **Tag her yellow and have someone sit with her one-to-one—YES, this is the best option if possible.**

Exercise 6-12: *Matching*

Match the designation in Column A with the patient condition in Column B; designations can be used more than once.

Column A		Column B
A. Morgue (Black)	**B**	Compound open femur fracture
B. Immediate (Red)	**C**	Burns over 20% of body from explosion
C. Delayed (Yellow)	**B**	Back injury, cannot feel legs
D. Minor (Green)	**B**	Debris in left eye
	B	Finger amputated
	B	Blunt trauma to abdomen, vomiting
	A	Crushed chest with perforated lungs
	B	Stroke

7

Ethics

Unfolding Case Study #7 Beyonce

Beyonce is scheduled for her second clinical leadership day with the nurse leader who is the chairperson of the hospital ethics committee as well as a patient liaison. She is very excited about this opportunity.

 eResource 7-1: To prepare for clinical, Beyonce
  ▓ Reviews a series of four videos: (1) *What Is Ethics?* (2) *5 Ways to Think Ethically*, (3) *Strategies to Manage Ethics*, and (4) *Am I Responsible?*: http://goo.gl/mkgRD
  ▓ In addition, Beyonce wants to make sure she has some readily available reference resources on her mobile device and finds the University of California School of Medicine's *Ethics Fast Facts*: http://goo.gl/6dx8L

The hospital ethics committee is meeting this afternoon, so Beyonce will be able to attend with her preceptor. Beyonce's preceptor greets her in the morning and asks Beyonce to help him prepare for the upcoming ethics case that will be discussed that afternoon at the ethics committee forum. The preceptor reviews some basic information about health care ethics with Beyonce first.

Exercise 7-1: *Matching*
Match the word in Column A to the definition in Column B.

Column A	Column B
A. Beneficence	_____ Keeping your word
B. Nonmaleficence	_____ Letting patients make their own decisions
C. Justice	_____ Duty to do good
D. Autonomy	_____ Telling the truth
E. Fidelity	_____ Respect for a patient's decision
F. Respect	_____ Fairness
G. Veracity	_____ Do no harm

eResource 7-2: Beyonce's preceptor explains that ethics is guided by different theories and that all nurses should understand the basis of the theories as well as read two important documents:

■ The American Nurses Association (ANA). (2001). *Code of Ethics for Nurses with Interpretive Statements*. Silver Spring, MD: ANA: http://goo.gl/mSPrD

■ The American Nurses Association (ANA). (2004). *Nursing's Social Policy Statement*. Washington, DC: ANA: http://goo.gl/PmFpP

The preceptor provides Beyonce with some theory examples.

Exercise 7-2: *Multiple-choice question*

A patient has varicella and is forced to stay in her room in order to reduce contamination of others. This demonstrates the ethical theory of:

    A. Utilitarianism

    B. Teleology

    C. Deontology

    D. Morality

Exercise 7-3: *Multiple-choice question*

A nurse helps her chemically addicted friend by supplying the friend with money for rent and food because she does not want to see the friend suffer. The friend uses the money for drugs. The nurse acted under the ethical theory of:

    A. Utilitarianism

    B. Teleology

    C. Deontology

    D. Morality

Exercise 7-4: *Multiple-choice question*

A nurse lets a family member into the intensive care unit to see her spouse after visiting hours because the person works late and cannot come during the normal hours. The family is happy and the unit workflow is not disrupted. The nurse used what ethical theory to make this decision?

    A. Utilitarianism

    B. Teleology

    C. Deontology

    D. Morality

Next the preceptor gives Beyonce questions about ethical principles that are commonly used in health care situations.

Answers to this chapter begin on page 99.

Exercise 7-5: *Multiple-choice question*

A patient is refusing chemotherapy and states she would rather die. The son is telling the patient that she does not have a choice and must take the chemotherapy. What statement by the nurse demonstrates autonomy?

> A. "Are you your mother's durable power of health care?"
> B. "I think you should consider your son's position."
> C. "Your mother has the right to decide if she wants chemotherapy."
> D. "Would you like to speak to your primary care provider about your decision?"

 eResource 7-3: To supplement her understanding of the concepts associated with ethical decision making, Beyonce refers to Santa Clara University's *Ethical Decision Making* web resource: http://goo.gl/ec7oq

Exercise 7-6: *Multiple-choice question*

A patient is admitted to the emergency department (ED) after an auto accident and asks the nurse "I was texting and driving; the accident was my fault. Do you know if my passenger is okay?" The nurse knows that the passenger is in critical condition. Using the ethical concept of veracity, how should the nurse answer?

> A. "I am not sure of your passenger's condition."
> B. "I can ask the ED primary care provider for you."
> C. "Your passenger is in critical condition."
> D. "You need to worry about yourself first, then we can deal with that."

 eResource 7-4: To reinforce her understanding of ethical philosophies and the responsibility of nurses, the preceptor shows Beyonce several videos:
> ▪ *Ethical Issues in Nursing—Respect: Dignity, Autonomy, and Relationships:* http://youtu.be/-GxuvKRL7ks
> ▪ *Ethical Issues in Nursing—Commitment: Patients, Professionalism, and Boundaries:* http://youtu.be/XtuanLybaZs

Beyonce states, "I can't think of any situation in which I would not be honest with a patient or family member. I think that would be a universal principle." The preceptor explains to Beyonce that situations change all the time and every situation is different.

Exercise 7-7: *Multiple-choice question*

A patient has died unexpectedly on the medical-surgical unit and the nurse needs to call the family. The patient's spouse answers the phone. The best response for the nurse is:

> A. "Please come to the hospital, your spouse has died."
> B. "Please come to the hospital, it is an emergency."
> C. "Please come to the hospital, your spouse has taken a turn for the worse."
> D. "Please come to the hospital now."

Answers to this chapter begin on page 99.

Beyonce understands the different theories and principles and asks her preceptor how they are all integrated during a committee decision about a real patient situation. Beyonce's preceptor explains the role of the ethics committee.

Exercise 7-8: *Select all that apply*
The role of a health care organization's ethics committee includes:
- ❑ Educating health care professionals about ethical principles
- ❑ Consultation for decision making for family
- ❑ Consultation for decision making for health care professionals
- ❑ Deciding on the appropriate patient option
- ❑ Providing a second health care opinion on cases
- ❑ Developing organizational policies

Beyonce's preceptor also tells her that he relies heavily on the *Code of Ethics for Nurses with Interpretive Statements* (2001).

Exercise 7-9: *Multiple-choice question*
According to the interpretive statements in the *Code of Ethics for Nurses*, the nurse's primary responsibility is to:
- A. Self
- B. Patient
- C. Patient and family
- D. Public

Beyonce's preceptor continues the discussion by explaining the decision processes that are involved when dealing with ethical dilemmas.

 eResource 7-5: To help Beyonce understand the decision process utilized when dealing with ethical dilemmas, he shows her *The ABCDE of Medical Ethics for Medical Students*: http://youtu.be/dGLcYVQeUAE

Exercise 7-10: *Multiple-choice question*
According to the interpretive statement the nurse "advocates," which means protecting:
- A. Ethical practice
- B. Interdisciplinary collaboration in care
- C. Patient rights
- D. Organizational functioning

 eResource 7-6: To supplement her understand of the decision-making process, Beyonce
- ▦ Views a brief video presentation *Tips to Improve the Decision Making Process:* http://goo.gl/guvW1
- ▦ Completes two learning activities:
  - ▦ Decision-Making Methods: http://goo.gl/rZ0Qo
  - ▦ Problem Solving and Decision Making: http://goo.gl/2MeAk

Answers to this chapter begin on page 99.

As Beyonce and her preceptor are talking, the nurse preceptor's phone rings. He is not only the nurse ethicist but a patient liaison and is often called for situations in which the staff nurses need assistance. A surgical nurse calls and requests him to come up to speak with a patient.

Exercise 7-11: *Multiple-choice question*
The patient states, "I do not want to have surgery again for my colon cancer. I am tired and just want to tie up the loose ends in my life while I can. I am being forced into this surgery." The best response to this statement would be:

    A. "Can you tell me what your major concern is about the surgery?"
    B. "The cancer will grow rapidly without the surgery."
    C. "No one can force you into having surgery."
    D. "Do you think a second opinion would help?"

 eResource 7-7: Beyonce quickly consults her mobile device to review information regarding a patient's rights to refuse treatment: http://goo.gl/JkPj8

The preceptor tell Beyonce that he is often called to help in impromptu situations and that the ethics committee members have to be ready to meet any time also. The committee comprises nurses, physicians, a respiratory therapist, hospital administrator, clergy, and a community person. Often families are invited to discuss the patient situation if appropriate.

Exercise 7-12: *Multiple-choice question*
The most frequent issues brought to the ethics committee have to do with:

    A. Perinatal
    B. Organ donation
    C. End of life
    D. Chemotherapy

After lunch the preceptor takes Beyonce to the ethics committee and the case is presented (Figure 7-1).

Figure 7-1: Case #1

Mr. A. is an 88-year-old male who was admitted for a head injury. He has an intracranial bleed and is initially confused and combative. After the active bleeding stops he is in a nonresponsive state. His family understands that he will probably not get better. He develops pneumonia and the decision is made to keep him comfortable. His daughter has durable power of health care and tells the residents to insert a feeding tube because "her father is not going to starve to death." The nurses on the unit brought this case to the ethics committee because it appears to them that it is in exact opposition of his living will, which states that he does not want any life-sustaining treatment.

Answers to this chapter begin on page 99.

Exercise 7-13: *Select all that apply*
Advance directives usually include:
- ❏ Living will statement
- ❏ Memorandum of understanding
- ❏ Durable power of attorney
- ❏ Organ donation
- ❏ Funeral preferences

The committee members discuss the case first and then ask the family members to join the discussion. While the health care providers were alone they discussed the ethical conflict.

Exercise 7-14: *Multiple-choice question*
The patient's daughter is acting under what ethical principle?
- A. Beneficence
- B. Justice
- C. Autonomy
- D. Veracity

The members of the ethics committee are concerned with the violation of the patient's written living will.

Exercise 7-15: *Multiple-choice question*
The members of the ethics committee are concerned specifically with which ethical principle?
- A. Beneficence
- B. Justice
- C. Autonomy
- D. Veracity

After the discussion the committee asks the family to come in and discuss their feelings about the situation with Mr. A. The family asks the physician present many questions about the prognosis and the time Mr. A would have left. The committee members bring up the issues of "quality of life" regarding Mr. A's condition. Mr. A's daughter is overtly upset and she is crying. The committee asks her to explain how she feels and she states that she does not want to lose her father and that she can't bear the thought of him dying. One of the committee members is a pastor and asks the daughter if she would like to discuss her feelings in private and she agrees. The committee disbands and will reconvene tomorrow after Mr. A's daughter has had time to discuss her feelings privately. Until then nothing different in Mr. A's care will be done.

After the meeting, Beyonce asks a lot of questions that the preceptor answers or provides resources for. Her first question has to do with the nurse's responsibility of living wills.

Answers to this chapter begin on page 99.

Exercise 7-16: *Multiple-choice question*

Nurses are responsible for which of the following interventions regarding advance directives?

❏ Ask all patients if they have an advance directive

❏ Assist all patients to make an advance directive

❏ Assist parents to make advance directives for children who are minors

❏ Provide the primary care provider with a copy of the advance directive

❏ Ensure the patient understands what is already on his or her advance directive

❏ Place the advance directive on the patient's chart or note it in the electronic medical record (EMR)

 eResource 7-8: Beyonce reviews a patient teaching video that explains *Advance Medical Directives* in simple terms: http://youtu.be/Hh8M-gx8Kt0

Mr. A's advance directive had a living will that stated that he did not want to be resuscitated if he stopped breathing or his heart stopped.

Exercise 7-17: *Multiple-choice question*

The preferred term for do not resuscitate (DNR) is:

❏ Comfort measures only

❏ Palliative care

❏ Expectant care

❏ Allow natural death (AND)

Exercise 7-18: *Multiple-choice question*

Beyonce asks the preceptor why a person needs a living will and a durable power of health care, and the preceptor correctly states:

A. "To ensure that everything in the living will is carried out"

B. "To determine if the living will should be followed"

C. "To override the living will if circumstances change or are unusual"

D. "To cover any circumstance that is not addressed in the living will"

 eResource 7-9: To learn more about advance directives, Beyonce reviews the topic in the University of California San Francisco's (UCSF) publication *Ethics Fast Facts:* http://goo.gl/uVme7

During their discussion the preceptor gets a call from the nurses on the medical unit who ask him to come and assist with a patient in his nurse liaison role. Beyonce and the preceptor go to the patient's room. The patient has complaints about the care received.

Answers to this chapter begin on page 99.

Exercise 7-19: *Multiple-choice question*

The patient tells Beyonce and the preceptor that he does not like his primary care provider.

How should the nurse respond to this statement?

    A. "Did you talk to the provider about this?"

    B. "Do you want me to talk to your provider?"

    C. "Tell me more about this."

    D. "Many people have complained about this provider."

 eResource 7-10: Beyonce watches the preceptor interacting with the patient and sees that he is using the techniques she read about in *Therapeutic Communication in Psychiatric Nursing*: http://goo.gl/UnCdX

After the nurse ethicist/liaison speaks with the patient for a while, the patient decides to get a second opinion. The nurse ethicist/liaison believes that this is a good solution for the patient and makes an appointment to follow up with him. The preceptor explains to Beyonce that he is called often to intervene in situations because many times the staff nurses do not have time to sit and talk things through with the patients and families. He said he was called just the other day for a "tough case."

A 32-year-old male who has two small children had been brought in the day before after a bad fall from a crane while working and is currently on a ventilator. The preceptor asks Beyonce a question about the situation.

Exercise 7-20: *Multiple-choice question*

The nurse caring for the patient on the ventilator just received word that the third electroencephalogram (EEG) demonstrated that there was no brain activity. What was the nurse's priority at this point in time?

    A. Request an order to remove the patient from the ventilator

    B. Call the organ donor team

    C. Request an MRI of the brain for confirmation

    D. Check the patient's advance directive for preferences

Beyonce asks the preceptor if he only takes care of patient issues. The preceptor answers that sometimes he is called to take care of staff dilemmas. He explains that he is a role model to the staff who are in situations with other staff that represent ethical dilemmas and tries to provide them with *moral courage* to do the right thing. One of the things he is often consulted on is chemical dependency of a staff member.

Exercise 7-21: *Multiple-choice question*

A nurse suspects a fellow nurse of diverting narcotics. What should the nurse do first?

    A. Approach the suspected nurse with the suspicion

    B. Take a picture of the activity for proof

    C. Report the suspicion to the hospital hotline

    D. Report the suspicion to the director

Answers to this chapter begin on page 99.

Other situations in which the preceptor has been involved are situations where a staff nurse needed support for showing moral courage and reporting instances that would place patients in danger. Beyonce is amazed at the many complex roles a nurse can have within a health care institution. Beyonce decides to stop back the following day after class to find out what happened with the case of Mr. A. Beyonce has permission to share the information about the case with her class without using any identifying data. Beyonce thanks her preceptor and leaves the clinical area for the day.

Answers to this chapter begin on page 99.

Answers

Exercise 7-1: *Matching*

Match the word in Column A to the definition in Column B.

Column A		Column B
A. Beneficence	__E__	Keeping your word
B. Nonmaleficence	__F__	Letting patients make their own decisions
C. Justice	__A__	Duty to do good
D. Autonomy	__G__	Telling the truth
E. Fidelity	__D__	Respect for a patient's decision
F. Respect	__C__	Fairness
G. Veracity	__B__	Do no harm

Exercise 7-2: *Multiple-choice question*

A patient has varicella and is forced to stay in her room in order to reduce contamination of others. This demonstrates the ethical theory of:

A. **Utilitarianism—YES, this provides the greatest good for the greatest number of people.**

B. Teleology—NO, in this theory the outcome matters most.

C. Deontology—NO, in this theory the process matters, not just the outcome.

D. Morality—NO, this is a general term for doing what is right.

Exercise 7-3: *Multiple-choice question*

A nurse helps her chemically addicted friend by supplying the friend with money for rent and food because she does not want to see the friend suffer. The friend uses the money for drugs. The nurse acted under the ethical theory of:

A. Utilitarianism—NO, this provides the greatest good for the greatest number of people.

B. Teleology—NO, in this theory the outcome matters most.

C. **Deontology—YES, in this theory the process matters, not just the outcome; the nurse was acting out of good will.**

D. Morality—NO, this is a general term for doing what is right.

Exercise 7-4: *Multiple-choice question*

A nurse lets a family member into the intensive care unit to see her spouse after visiting hours because the person works late and cannot come during the normal hours. The family is happy and the unit workflow is not disrupted. The nurse used what ethical theory to make this decision?

A. Utilitarianism—NO, this provides the greatest good for the greatest number of people.

B. **Teleology—YES, in this theory the outcome matters most.**

C. Deontology—NO, in this theory the process matters, not just the outcome.

D. Morality—NO, this is a general term for doing what is right.

Exercise 7-5: *Multiple-choice question*

A patient is refusing chemotherapy and states she would rather die. The son is telling the patient that she does not have a choice and must take the chemotherapy. What statement by the nurse demonstrates autonomy?

A. "Are you your mother's durable power of health care?"—NO, this is known by the documentation on the chart.

B. "I think you should consider your son's position."—NO, this is bullying the patient.

C. **"Your mother has the right to decide if she wants chemotherapy."—YES, this is the best response to be an advocate and promote autonomy for the patient.**

D. "Would you like to speak to your primary care provider about your decision?"—NO, this will not address the problem at hand.

Exercise 7-6: *Multiple-choice question*

A patient is admitted to the emergency department (ED) after an auto accident and asks the nurse "I was texting and driving; the accident was my fault. Do you know if my passenger is okay?" The nurse knows that the passenger is in critical condition. Using the ethical concept of veracity, how should the nurse answer?

A. "I am not sure of your passenger's condition."—NO, this is not telling the truth.

B. "I can ask the ED primary care provider for you."—NO, this is not telling the truth.

C. **"Your passenger is in critical condition."—YES, this is telling the truth.**

D. "You need to worry about yourself first, then we can deal with that."—NO, this is not telling the truth.

Exercise 7-7: *Multiple-choice question*

A patient has died unexpectedly on the medical-surgical unit and the nurse needs to call the family. The patient's spouse answers the phone. The best response for the nurse is:

A. "Please come to the hospital, your spouse has died."—NO, this does not consider the person's safety because he or she has to drive to the hospital.

B. "Please come to the hospital, it is an emergency."—NO, this leaves unanswered questions and will prompt the person to ask them.

C. **"Please come to the hospital, your spouse has taken a turn for the worse."—YES, this denotes urgency and even though it does not tell the whole truth, it may place the driver in less danger on the road.**

D. "Please come to the hospital now."—NO, this leaves unanswered questions and will prompt the person to ask them.

Exercise 7-8: *Select all that apply*
The role of a health care organization's ethics committee includes:

☒ **Educating health care professionals about ethical principles—YES, this is a role.**

☒ **Consultation for decision making for family—YES, this is a role.**

☒ **Consultation for decision making for health care professionals—YES, this is a role.**

☐ Deciding on the appropriate patient option—NO, they do not tell people or professionals what to do.

☐ Providing a second health care opinion on cases—NO, they do not tell people or professionals what to do.

☒ **Developing organizational policies—YES, this is a role.**

Exercise 7-9: *Multiple-choice question*
According to the interpretive statements in the *Code of Ethics for Nurses*, the nurse's primary responsibility is to:

A. Self—NO

B. **Patient—YES**

C. Patient and family—NO

D. Public—NO

Exercise 7-10: *Multiple-choice question*
According to the interpretive statement the nurse "advocates," which means protecting:

A. Ethical practice—NO

B. Interdisciplinary collaboration in care—NO

C. **Patient rights—YES**

D. Organizational functioning—NO

Exercise 7-11: *Multiple-choice question*
The patient states, "I do not want to have surgery again for my colon cancer. I am tired and just want to tie up the loose ends in my life while I can. I am being forced into this surgery." The best response to this statement would be:

A. "Can you tell me what your major concern is about the surgery?"—NO, this is undermining the patient by prolonging the issue.

B. "The cancer will grow rapidly without the surgery."—NO, this is threatening.

C. **"No one can force you into having surgery."—YES, this is appropriately being an advocate.**

D. "Do you think a second opinion would help?"—NO, this is undermining the patient by persuasion.

Exercise 7-12: *Multiple-choice question*
The most frequent issues brought to the ethics committee have to do with:

A. Perinatal—NO, although there are many perinatal ethical issues.

B. Organ donation—NO

C. **End of life—YES**

D. Chemotherapy—NO

Exercise 7-13: *Select all that apply*
Advance directives usually include:

☒ **Living will statement—YES, this is one part of an advance directive.**

☐ Memorandum of understanding—NO, this is not a part of the document.

☐ Durable power of attorney—NO, a durable power of health care is part of the document.

☐ Organ donation—NO, this is on people's drivers' licenses.

☐ Funeral preferences—NO

Exercise 7-14: *Multiple-choice question*
The patient's daughter is acting under what ethical principle?

A. **Beneficence—YES, she is trying to do good.**

B. Justice—NO, there is no real fairness issue.

C. Autonomy—NO

D. Veracity—NO

Exercise 7-15: *Multiple-choice question*
The members of the ethics committee are concerned specifically with which ethical principle?

A. Beneficence—NO, this is not the primary concern at this point.

B. Justice—NO, fairness is not the primary concern at this point.

C. **Autonomy—YES, the patient's ability to make his own decisions.**

D. Veracity—NO, truth is not the primary concern at this point.

Exercise 7-16: *Multiple-choice question*
Nurses are responsible for which of the following interventions regarding advance directives:

☒ **Ask all patients if they have an advance directive—YES, nurses should ask every patient if he or she has an advance directive.**

☐ Assist all patients to make an advance directive—NO, if they need one, they are usually referred to the legal department or a case worker.

❏ Assist parents to make advance directives for children who are minors—NO, this is not the nurse's job.

❏ Provide the primary care provider with a copy of the advance directive—NO, they can find it on the chart.

❏ Ensure the patient understands what is already on his or her advance directive—NO, this was done when it was made.

☒ **Place the advance directive on the patient's chart or note it in the electronic medical record (EMR)—YES, it must be placed in the chart.**

Exercise 7-17: *Multiple-choice question*

The preferred term for do not resuscitate (DNR) is:

❏ Comfort measures only—NO

❏ Palliative care—NO

❏ Expectant care—NO

☒ **Allow natural death (AND)—YES, AND is a better term for families because it does not denote they are taking or withholding something like DNR sounds.**

Exercise 7-18: *Multiple-choice question*

Beyonce asks the preceptor why a person needs a living will and a durable power of health care, and the preceptor correctly states:

A. "To ensure that everything in the living will is carried out"—NO, this is not the reason because things are written down and legally and ethically need to be followed.

B. "To determine if the living will should be followed"—NO, this is not the reason because things are written down and legally and ethically need to be followed.

C. "To override the living will if circumstances change or are unusual"—NO, this is not the reason because things are written down and legally and ethically need to be followed.

D. **"To cover any circumstance that is not addressed in the living will"—YES, not everything can be anticipated.**

Exercise 7-19: *Multiple-choice question*

The patient tells Beyonce and the preceptor that he does not like his primary care provider.

How should the nurse respond to this statement?

A. "Did you talk to the provider about this?"—NO, that is not dealing with the patient's strong feelings.

B. "Do you want me to talk to your provider?"—NO, that is not dealing with the patient's strong feelings.

C. **"Tell me more about this."—YES, this opens up the discussion for better understanding.**

D. "Many people have complained about this provider."—NO, this is professionally inappropriate.

Exercise 7-20: *Multiple-choice question*

The nurse caring for the patient on the ventilator just received word that the third electroencephalogram (EEG) demonstrated that there was no brain activity. What was the nurse's priority at this point in time?

  A. Request an order to remove the patient from the ventilator—NO, this is not the priority yet.
  B. **Call the organ donor team—YES**
  C. Request an MRI of the brain for confirmation—NO, this is not needed; there is a definitive diagnosis with three flat EEGs.
  D. Check the patient's advance directive for preferences—NO, the patient is legally dead and needs to be taken off the ventilator.

Exercise 7-21: *Multiple-choice question*

A nurse suspects a fellow nurse of diverting narcotics. What should the nurse do first?

  A. Approach the suspected nurse with the suspicion—NO, this will most likely produce denial from the suspect.
  B. Take a picture of the activity for proof—NO, this is invading privacy.
  C. Report the suspicion to the hospital hotline—NO, this is usually used when middle management is unresponsive.
  D. **Report the suspicion to the director—YES, this is the first chain of command and ethically the right thing to do.**

8

Health Care Informatics

Linda Wilson and Frances H. Cornelius

Unfolding Case Study #8 ▨ Roxanne

Roxanne also had a leadership clinical experience this week and was precepted by the hospital informatics nurse. The informatics nurse has a very interesting hospital job and is a key person in the organization. The informatics nurse maintains staff education on system updates, communicates important information systemwide, and runs hospital-wide interdisciplinary simulation scenarios. Roxanne meets the informatics nurse in the morning and they review the day's agenda. First they will check on the medical-surgical unit's electronic health records (EHRs) management. The medical-surgical unit just went "live" last week and was the last unit to begin using the EHR system. Now the system is fully integrated into the hospital. After visiting the medical-surgical unit they will upgrade the nursing minimum data set (NMDS) to include some new nursing diagnoses.

 eResource 8-1: Roxanne reviews the information regarding NMDS from the University of Minnesota Center for Nursing Informatics: [Pathway: http://goo.gl/ZtTDt → review content "i-NMDS," "USA NMDS," and "USA NMMDS"]

After lunch they will check on staff competencies that are now done by computer tutorial and then run an interdisciplinary simulation. Roxanne is excited to get the day started and her preceptor provides her with some background information about health information systems. "Two terms that are often used interchangeably are electronic medical records (EMRs) and electronic health records (EHRs). In truth, they are not the same. EMRs are more 'clinically focused' for the purpose of diagnosis and treatment while the EHR is a more encompassing, broader system that has a broader view on the patient and the patient's care—going beyond standard clinical data collected in an EMR."

Exercise 8-1: *Multiple-choice question*
The Department of Health and Human Services' (DHHS) goal for EHR is:

    A. Have all health care organizations up and running by 2020

Answers to this chapter begin on page 111.   **105**

B. Have all patients in the United States have a specific bar code on their license to identify them in the system

C. Connect all health care systems to a national database

D. Develop a national health care worker database so people can work easily in underserved areas

 eResource 8-2: To learn more about the EHR Incentive Programs, Roxanne visits CMS.gov: [Pathway: www.cms.gov → enter "EHR" into the search field → select "EHR incentive program" and review content]

Exercise 8-2: *Select all that apply*

EHRs should contain the following information:

❑ Biographical data

❑ Past medical history

❑ Criminal charges

❑ Foreign travel

❑ Nursing diagnosis

❑ Social history

Exercise 8-3: *Multiple-choice question*

The Institute of Medicine (IOM) wants EHRs in place within 10 years to use the collective data for research on:

A. Patient satisfaction

B. Cost containment

C. Health profession burnout

D. Patient safety

 eResource 8-3: To learn more about the benefits of EHRs, Roxanne visits HealthIT.gov: [Pathway: www.healthit.gov → enter "Benefits of EHR" into the search field → select "Benefits of Electronic Health Records (EHRs)" and review content]

On the medical-surgical unit Roxanne and her preceptor find that most of the staff are adjusting to the EHR system but with some frustrations, which is to be expected. Maneuvering around in the system takes time to get used to and management in the organization has anticipated this reaction.

Exercise 8-4: *Select all that apply*

Some proactive leadership interventions that can assist staff to get used to a new process include:

❑ Having resources present on the unit

❑ Telling them they can revert back to the old system if frustrated

❑ Watching each of them enter data for a day

Answers to this chapter begin on page 111.

❏ Having an informational technology (IT) specialist on the hotline from 7 a.m. to 7 p.m.

❏ Educating them as they get into the process

❏ Increase staffing levels

eResource 8-4: The preceptor shares with Roxanne the step-by-step process used to plan the EHR implementation process: [Pathway: www.healthit.gov → enter "implementation EHR" into the search field → select "How to Implement EHRs" and review content]

Roxanne watches her preceptor explain to a nurse how to get from the admission screen to the lab screen and to open up the lab values so that they can be checked against the normal values. Another staff nurse is having difficulty scanning a patient's armband in order to give a medication. The nurse is using the Medication Administration Record (MAR) within the EHR.

Exercise 8-5: *Multiple-choice question*

The nurse administering medications understands the MAR when the nurse states:

    A. "I can give the medication so it will not be late until the resource IT person can help me."

    B. "The medication can be overridden in the system so it is not administered late."

    C. "The arm band is wet and needs to be changed so I can give the medication."

    D. "The patient can provide two identifiers so I can administer the medication and manually mark it in the computer."

Roxanne asks the preceptor about the EHR and the medication orders. The preceptor tells her that medication orders are entered into the system using CPOE and once entered, a flag pops up on the screen to notify the person who is working in the system and is responsible for administering medications.

Exercise 8-6: *Multiple-choice question*

CPOE stands for:

    A. Computerized pharmacy order entry

    B. Custom pharmacy order entry

    C. Computerized physician/order entry

    D. Computer physician order entry

Exercise 8-7: *Select all that apply*

The secondary purposes of EHRs include:

    ❏ Education

    ❏ Patient care delivery

    ❏ Financial processes

    ❏ Research

    ❏ Homeland security

    ❏ Regulation

Answers to this chapter begin on page 111.

After Roxanne and her preceptor finish assisting staff by troubleshooting the EHR, the preceptor tells Roxanne that this support function is important not only at this time, but must be sustained over time.

 eResource 8-5: As the preceptor explains that long-term support is essential to the successful implementation of the EHR, Roxanne remembers that in class, a guest speaker had discussed *EMR Implementation Challenges*: http://goo.gl/18i0L

Roxanne realizes that the same challenges of EHR implementation described by the guest speaker are experienced with implementation of broader EHR systems as well. Just as Roxanne and her preceptor finish this conversation, the elevator door opens and a robot rolls off. The robot is from central supply and is delivering supplies to the nursing care unit. It works by being pre-programmed and navigates with a sensor.

Roxanne also observes a nurse using a mobile device to look up medication side effects. Roxanne asks her preceptor about nurses using smartphones for information retrieval while at work.

Exercise 8-8: *Multiple-choice question*

The best policy for the use of smartphones includes:

    A. Not using them at all due to breaches in the Health Insurance Portability and Accountability Act (HIPAA)

    B. Only using them in the patient's room

    C. Using them for needed health care resources only

    D. Keeping your patient information on them

After lunch Roxanne and her preceptor go to the simulation lab for an interdisciplinary simulation event. The event involves a multidisciplinary team that includes medical personnel, nursing, respiratory therapists, and unlicensed assistive personnel. The scenario was a patient case scenario (Figure 8-1).

Figure 8-1:   Patient Case Scenario

I	I am Linda, GN, working in the emergency department and taking care of Mr. H.
S	Mr. H is a 68-year-old patient who was mowing his lawn on a ride-on mower when he got stung by a bee.
B	Mr. H. has chronic obstructive pulmonary disease (COPD) and hypertension. He was a smoker for 30 years but quit 8 years ago. He is on Spiriva daily and Lipitor.
A	The patient appears to be having a reaction to the bee sting and is complaining of his throat "feeling tight." He has a rash on his face, trunk, and neck that is bright red and one of his eyes is swollen.
R	
R	

Answers to this chapter begin on page 111.

Exercise 8-9: *Multiple-choice question*
Roxanne is invited to participate in the simulation and is assigned the RN role in the case scenario. Roxanne's priority care in this simulated situation would be:

    A. Administer oxygen at 8 L/min via nasal cannula

    B. Call the emergency department (ED) physician for Benadryl IM

    C. Call the in-house anesthesiologist to intubate Mr. H

    D. Call the rapid response team (RRT)

Roxanne assists the team by drawing medication and retrieving equipment. The team is working together on the patient. The registered respiratory therapist assesses air exchange and determines that the patient's airway needs to be protected and suggests intubation. The ED physician intubates and then Roxanne starts an intravenous line. Benadryl is given intravenously and the patient is placed on minimal oxygen due to his COPD. He is also placed on a cardio-respiratory (C-R) monitor for a constant vital sign and pulse oximetry read out. The patient is stabilized and the team transports him to an intensive care unit (ICU) bed.

Exercise 8-10: *Multiple-choice question*
To complete the I-SBAR-R communication tool, which response would be best?

    A. The patient was stabilized and moved to an ICU bed for close observation

    B. The patient did well once intubated and maintained a pulse oxygen of 96%

    C. The patient is in critical condition at this point but is expected to get better

    D. The patient now needs to wear a Medi Alert bracelet for bee stings because he had such a severe reaction

> **eResource 8-6:** Roxanne recalls a lecture regarding effective communication using SBAR:
> - Using SBAR: http://goo.gl/RJvtf
> - SBAR: Effective Communication:
>   - Example 1: http://goo.gl/yHx8O
>   - Example 2: http://goo.gl/RE3fi

During the debriefing, Roxanne watches the video of the event with the team. Roxanne realizes that there are some things that may have been done differently.

Exercise 8-11: *Multiple-choice question*
The main purpose of debriefing is to:

    A. Remediate

    B. Reflect

    C. Have a basis to redo

    D. Reinforce

Answers to this chapter begin on page 111.

Exercise 8-12: *Multiple-choice question*

During a debriefing, a simulation participant can expect:

     A. A grade

     B. Clinical evaluation checklist

     C. Rigorous feedback with genuine inquiry

     D. A pass/fail

Roxanne finds the debriefing helpful and many of the participants talk about how much they learned from watching themselves. One of the participants in the debriefing session said she felt herself getting upset as if it were a real patient.

Exercise 8-13: *Multiple-choice question*

Simulated experiences are organized and developed in order to:

     A. Bridge the gap between classroom and clinical experiences

     B. Take the place of all clinical experiences

     C. Demonstrate if a student or nurse is ready to care for patients

     D. Decide if patients with high acuity can be cared for safely

Roxanne has learned a tremendous amount today about EHR and simulation and is very thankful to her preceptor. She can't wait to get back to class to tell her colleagues about how important technology is for safe patient care.

Answers to this chapter begin on page 111.

Answers

Exercise 8-1: *Multiple-choice question*

The Department of Health and Human Services' (DHHS) goal for EHR is:

   A. Have all health care organizations up and running by 2020—NO, although this would be an asset, it is not the complete goal.

   B. Have all patients in the United States have a specific bar code on their license to identify them in the system—NO, this too may be an asset but many people do not have a driver's license.

   C. **Connect all health care systems to a national database—YES, this is the goal.**

   D. Develop a national health care worker database so people can work easily in underserved areas—NO, although data collected may be able to be used in this manner

Exercise 8-2: *Select all that apply*

EHRs should contain the following information:

☒ **Biographical data—YES**

☒ **Past medical history—YES**

☐ Criminal charges—NO, this is not a necessary health care piece of information.

☒ **Foreign travel—YES**

☒ **Nursing diagnosis—YES**

☒ **Social history—YES**

Exercise 8-3: *Multiple-choice question*

The Institute of Medicine (IOM) wants EHRs in place within 10 years to use the collective data for research on:

   A. Patient satisfaction—NO, this is not the goal.

   B. Cost containment—NO, this is not the goal.

   C. Health profession burnout—NO, this is not the goal.

   D. **Patient safety—YES, this is the ultimate goal of EHRs.**

Exercise 8-4: *Select all that apply*
Some proactive leadership interventions that can assist staff to get used to a new process include:

☒ **Having resources present on the unit—YES, troubleshooting as difficulties are developing is a great method by which to learn.**

☐ Telling them they can revert back to the old system if frustrated—NO, this does not help people learn a new system.

☐ Watching each of them enter data for a day—NO, this does not promote autonomy.

☒ **Having an informational technology (IT) specialist on the hotline from 7 a.m. to 7 p.m.—YES, troubleshooting as difficulties are developing is a great method by which to learn.**

☐ Educating them as they get into the process—NO, educating before the process is more effective.

☒ **Increase staffing levels—YES, this decreases the staff's feeling of being rushed.**

Exercise 8-5: *Multiple-choice question*
The nurse administering medications understands the MAR when the nurse states:
  A. "I can give the medication so it will not be late until the resource IT person can help me."—NO, the medication must be scanned to verify that it is correct.
  B. "The medication can be overridden in the system so it is not administered late."—NO, the medication must be scanned to verify that it is correct.
  C. **"The arm band is wet and needs to be changed so I can give the medication."—YES, this will allow the medication to be scanned to verify that it is correct.**
  D. "The patient can provide two identifiers so I can administer the medication and manually mark it in the computer."—NO, the medication must be scanned to verify that it is correct.

Exercise 8-6: *Multiple-choice question*
CPOE stands for:
  A. Computerized pharmacy order entry—NO
  B. Custom pharmacy order entry—NO
  C. Computerized physician/order entry –NO
  D. **Computer physician order entry—YES**

Exercise 8-7: *Select all that apply*
The secondary purposes of EHRs include:

☒ **Education—YES**

☐ Patient care delivery—NO, this is a primary purpose.

☐ Financial processes—NO, this is a primary purpose.

☒ **Research—YES**

☒ **Homeland security—YES**

☒ **Regulation—YES**

Exercise 8-8: *Multiple-choice question*
The best policy for the use of smartphones includes:
- A. Not using them at all due to breaches in the Health Insurance Portability and Accountability Act (HIPAA)—NO, they can be a valuable resource.
- B. Only using them in the patient's room—NO, this may not be appropriate.
- C. **Using them for needed health care resources only—YES**
- D. Keeping your patient information on them—NO, never; this is a HIPAA violation.

Exercise 8-9: *Multiple-choice question*
Roxanne is invited to participate in the simulation and is assigned the RN role in the case scenario. Roxanne's priority care in this simulated situation would be:
- A. Administer oxygen at 8 L/min via nasal cannula—NO, this is too much oxygen for a patient with COPD.
- B. Call the emergency department (ED) physician for Benadryl IM—NO, this does not protect the airway fast enough.
- C. Call the in-house anesthesiologist to intubate Mr. H—NO, this does not get people there quickly.
- D. **Call the rapid response team (RRT)—YES, this summons people quickly.**

Exercise 8-10: *Multiple-choice question*
To complete the I-SBAR-R communication tool, which response would be best?
- A. The patient was stabilized and moved to an ICU bed for close observation—NO, stabilized is a vague description.
- B. **The patient did well once intubated and maintained a pulse oxygen of 96%—YES, this gives some specific information.**
- C. The patient is in critical condition at this point but is expected to get better—NO, this cannot be predicted.
- D. The patient now needs to wear a Medi Alert bracelet for bee stings because he had such a severe reaction—NO, this is discharge information.

Exercise 8-11: *Multiple-choice question*
The main purpose of debriefing is to:
- A. Remediate—NO, this is not the objective of debriefing.
- B. **Reflect—YES, have the participants take a look at what they did well and what needs improvement.**
- C. Have a basis to redo—NO, this is not the objective of debriefing.
- D. Reinforce—NO, this is not the objective of debriefing.

Exercise 8-12: *Multiple-choice question*

During a debriefing, a simulation participant can expect:

A. A grade—NO, this is not always the goal.

B. Clinical evaluation checklist—NO, this is not always the goal.

C. **Rigorous feedback with genuine inquiry—YES, rigorous feedback with genuine inquiry is important regardless if the experience is one of learning or evaluation.**

D. A pass/fail—NO, this is not always the goal.

Exercise 8-13: *Multiple-choice question*

Simulated experiences are organized and developed in order to:

A. **Bridge the gap between classroom and clinical experiences—YES, this is the purpose.**

B. Take the place of all clinical experiences—NO, this is not the purpose of simulation.

C. Demonstrate if a student or nurse is ready to care for patients—NO, this is not the purpose of simulation.

D. Decide if patients with high acuity can be cared for safely—NO, this is not the purpose of simulation.

9

Nursing Unit Management

Unfolding Case Study #9 ▨ Jacob

At the next session Dr. Bennett has Roxanne and Beyonce tell the class about their clinical experiences. Beyonce also provides a follow-up to the ethical case that she was involved with.

After personal counseling, Mr. A's daughter consented to not start total parenteral nutrition (TPN) and to honor his living will. She was still distraught but held onto the notion that "this is what he would have wanted." The pastor counseled her about what "allow natural death" (AND) really means and that people are not in pain if feeding is withheld at the end of life. The learners thought the case was extremely interesting and many of them volunteered how they would have handled the situation if they were in a leadership position like the ethicist/liaison nurse.

 eResource 9-1: To supplement their understanding regarding this important topic, the class reviewed:
- ▨ *Approaching Death: Improving Care at the End of Life*: http://goo.gl/VoTwl
- ▨ The American College of Physicians' *ACP Ethics Manual, Sixth Edition*: [Pathway: http://goo.gl/5qvPt → scroll down and select "Care of Patients Near the End of Life" and review content]

The current class session has to do with nursing unit management issues that learners will most likely encounter soon after they are out of school. Unit management issues have to do with patients and staff as well as the work environment. The class outcomes are to discuss all three domains of nursing unit management.

eResource 9-2: To supplement the discussion, the class reads:
- ▨ *Functions of Administration in Nursing*: http://goo.gl/b2Zu1
- ▨ Nurse Manager Skills Inventory: http://goo.gl/33l80
- ▨ Nurse Unit Manager Role: http://goo.gl/nSvc4

Patient care is discussed first and has measurable outcomes.

Answers to this chapter begin on page 125.

Exercise 9-1: *Multiple-choice question*

Core measures are outcome data mandated of health care organizations by which agency?

      A. National Patient Safety Goals

      B. The Joint Commission

      C. Centers for Disease Control and Prevention

      D. Agency for Healthcare Research and Quality

Understanding core measures and nurse-sensitive indicators is important because they are patient safety issues and are reportable. A secondary issue that all nurses need to understand is the cost of health care.

Exercise 9-2: *Select all that apply*

A core measure for pneumonia is measured by the following actions:

      ❑ Coughing, turning, and deep breathing patients every 2 hours

      ❑ Providing antibiotics within 4 hours of admission

      ❑ Ensuring respiratory therapy is consulted

      ❑ Mouth care

      ❑ Acting on the information from cultures

      ❑ Decreasing suctioning

e   **eResource 9-3:** To learn more about core measures, the class visits The Joint Commission's website: [Pathway: www.jointcommission.org → enter "core measures" into the search field → select "Core Measure Sets" and review content]

Jacob asks Dr. Bennett how nurses are responsible for the financial aspects of patient care. Dr. Bennett tells him they are responsible in several ways. Cost containment includes many variables such as appropriate referrals, preventing complications, having an organized system so length of stay (LOS) is not prolonged, and increasing patient satisfaction so other patients want to come to the institution. Dr. Bennett gives the class some audience response system (ARS) questions to drive home the point.

Exercise 9-3: *Multiple-choice question*

The case manager notifies the primary care provider (PCP), who is in surgery, that the patient's insurance will not pay for another day's stay. What should the case manager do?

      A. Call the family to pick the patient up

      B. Notify the nursing supervisor of the situation

      C. Ask accounting to change the patient's status to nonpay

      D. Wait for the primary care provider

Answers to this chapter begin on page 125.

Exercise 9-4: *Multiple-choice question*

A patient has a neck injury and is unable to swallow well. What interdisciplinary intervention should the nurse include in the patient's care plan?

    A. Ask the family to bring protein shakes

    B. Ask the doctor for TPN

    C. Request a dietitian referral

    D. Request an occupational therapy referral

Exercise 9-5: *Multiple-choice question*

The nurse on a pediatric unit has a patient for the second time, an 8-year-old girl. The nurse remembers asking the parents to have the child's eyes checked because the child sits so close to the television and the parents have not followed through. The nurse should:

    A. Discuss the importance of eye exams

    B. Ask the PCP for a referral

    C. Get a family history of eye disorders

    D. Find out if they can afford the care

Exercise 9-6: *Multiple-choice question*

An emergency department (ED) nurse takes a report on three patients. One patient is a 24-hour observe and it is hour 23. The best action for the nurse would be:

    A. Discharge the patient

    B. Call the PCP to discharge the patient

    C. Transfer the patient to an inpatient unit and status

    D. Wait to see if the PCP makes round this shift

Exercise 9-7: *Multiple-choice question*

The nurse is discharging a postpartum patient who has a flat affect and a history of postpartum depression (PPD). Which is the appropriate referral?

    A. Primary care office

    B. PPD support group

    C. Mother and infant play group

    D. Mental health counselor

The learners now understand that prudent nursing care and practice decrease hospital costs, which are a concern in today's economy. The class takes a break and when they come back they talk about staffing on a nursing unit and managing a nursing unit's census. They are already familiar with the types of nursing care delivery systems but know that no matter what system is used—team, functional, primary, or total patient care—there are staffing issues with each.

 eResource 9-4: The class reviews an overview of staffing a unit by reading *Staffing in Nursing Units*: http://goo.gl/We3b8

Answers to this chapter begin on page 125.

Beyonce tells the class about an occurrence on the medical-surgical unit she was on last semester as a first-semester senior student. Beyonce heard a staff nurse complain about the night shift to the nurse manager.

Exercise 9-8: *Multiple-choice question*

A day-shift nurse complains to the unit director that the night shift never gets their work done and now the day shift is behind. The best response by the unit director is:

    A. "I will talk to them."
    B. "They usually do their best but must have gotten busy."
    C. "You should call a group meeting."
    D. "Provide me with examples of what you mean."

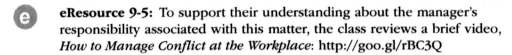 **eResource 9-5:** To support their understanding about the manager's responsibility associated with this matter, the class reviews a brief video, *How to Manage Conflict at the Workplace*: http://goo.gl/rBC3Q

Patient satisfaction reports are very important to a health care organization and reflect directly back on the culture of the patient care unit and the work environment produced by the team. Scores on patient satisfaction surveys are reportable to the Centers for Medicare and Medicaid Services (CMS) if the health care organization receives patient reimbursement from Medicare and Medicaid.

Exercise 9-9: *Multiple-choice question*

The lowest percent of patients that needs to be surveyed about satisfaction post discharge for reimbursement is:

    A. 5%
    B. 10%
    C. 25%
    D. 50%

Exercise 9-10: *Select all that apply*

The most important information collected on patient satisfaction surveys normally includes the following:

    ❑ Accessibility to care
    ❑ Communication skills of all providers
    ❑ Quality of care provided
    ❑ Dietary, lab, testing, and valet parking services
    ❑ Appearance of health care providers
    ❑ Facilities' quality

eResource 9-6: Dr. Bennett tells the class about an additional resource that provides information regarding care received in the hospital via a nonprofit organization called the Leap Frog Group, which provides a report card to the public on safety, quality, and affordability of

Answers to this chapter begin on page 125.

health care at participating health care organizations: [Pathway: www.leapfroggroup.org → scroll down and select "Hospital Safety Score" and "Compare Hospitals Now"]

The class seems to understand the importance of patient surveys, which then developed into a class discussion about work environment. Jacob asked, "What are the variables that create a positive work environment as opposed to a negative one?" Dr. Bennett provides some variables that could determine the work environment. He named issues such as interdisciplinary communication, leadership and self-governance, mentorship of new staff, patient-to-nurse ratios, pay, equity in scheduling, evaluations of staff, and competency testing. The class was over but Jacob's next clinical day was tomorrow and he was following the nurse manager of the ED at the largest hospital in town.

The following day Jacob meets the manager, who is called the director of the ED, and she orients him to the unit. The director explains to Jacob that she is responsible for staffing, scheduling, organizing, directing, budgeting, controlling, evaluating and hiring staff, and decision making. In the afternoon she is willing to have Jacob sit in on a monthly staff meeting.

Exercise 9-11: *Multiple-choice question*
First-level managers are responsible for unit operations:
    A. During the day shift while they are there
    B. If it pertains to specific issues only on that unit
    C. 24/7
    D. When the leader of all critical care units is off

The director also tells Jacob that she intervenes in patient care when needed. The ED is a very busy place and has a triage and fast-track room as well as 12 bays inside the ED. Two of the bays are held for psychiatric patients because they are more secluded at the end of the hall and there are less environmental stimuli in the area. One of the staff nurses calls the director in to talk to a patient with her.

Exercise 9-12: *Multiple-choice question*
A 16-year-old is in Bay 4 and has been told she has gonorrhea. She is crying and wants reassurance that no one will find out about this condition. The nurse's best response to the patient is:
    A. "You must tell your sexual partners so they can get treated."
    B. "You should tell your parents because they are going to see the health care bill."
    C. "Due to Health Insurance Portability and Accountability Act (HIPAA) regulations the information will be kept confidential."
    D. "Gonorrhea is a reportable disease to the Public Health Department."

As soon as they leave Bay 4, after speaking to the patient, Jacob and the director find an elderly patient wandering in the hall.

Answers to this chapter begin on page 125.

Exercise 9-13: *Multiple-choice question*

A patient being admitted for worsening dementia and urinary tract infection is wandering in the hall and states, "I am looking for the 5 and 10 cent store to buy a candy bar." The nurse's best response is:

    A. "I will show you where the store is" and leads the patient back to his bay.

    B. "This is the ED of a hospital, not the 5 and 10 cent store."

    C. "Let's talk about why you need to go to the store."

    D. "Let me help you back to your bed."

Jacob is concerned that this will happen again and the elderly gentlemen will wander out of the hospital.

Exercise 9-14: *Multiple-choice question*

The best nursing intervention for this patient with dementia would be:

    A. Restrain him

    B. Place him in a bay close to the nurses' station

    C. Call the family to sit with him

    D. Call the supervisor to get him on a locked unit

 eResource 9-7: To reinforce his understanding of the regulations, Jacob does a quick check for The Joint Commission's regulations on his smartphone: [Pathway: http://goo.gl/cwZ87 → select "JCAHO and CMS—Patient rights and use of restraints" and review summary]

A nurse calls out to the director for help in Bay 10. When Jacob and the director arrive in Bay 10, they find the following.

Exercise 9-15: *Multiple-choice question*

The patient in Bay 10 is diaphoretic and on the floor. He is ashen in color and states he just passed out but doesn't know why and feels like he has pain in his arm. The first thing the nurse should do is:

    A. Call the rapid response team

    B. Give him oxygen

    C. Get him back on the stretcher

    D. Get an electrocardiogram

After the patient in Bay 10 is cared for, a loud verbal squabble breaks out in the triage area of the ED. Jacob and the director respond.

Exercise 9-16: *Multiple-choice question*

A patient is brought in to the ED and is accompanied by his friends who are intoxicated. What should the nurse do?

    A. Call 911

    B. Call the local police

    C. Tell them to leave

    D. Call security

Answers to this chapter begin on page 125.

The director takes Jacob to her office to go over some staff issues and policies and procedures. She tells Jacob that she can spend all day "putting out fires" if she does not make time for the work she is responsible for. She also tells him that she is a democratic leader and that her staff knows she has an open-door policy if they need anything. The director tells Jacob that the staff schedule is developed on 4-week rotations of 12-hour shifts.

Exercise 9-17: *Multiple-choice question*
A democratic director would most likely adhere to:
    A. Block scheduling that is consistent for each schedule
    B. Staff self-scheduling
    C. Centralized scheduling
    D. Taking scheduling requests and trying to honor them

The director tells Jacob that she uses several experienced per-diem nurses on her unit, especially on the weekends when patient census is highest.

Exercise 9-18: *Select all that apply*
Advantages to working per diem instead of full time are:
    ❏ Consistent hours
    ❏ Lack of health benefits
    ❏ Flexible scheduling
    ❏ Most complex patient load
    ❏ Paid vacation time
    ❏ Not working major holidays

After lunch the scheduled staff meeting takes place and Jacob is invited to attend. Most of the day staff is present and six representatives from the night staff. The director has an agenda that deals with overall unit processes such as budget, patient survey results, and scheduling, and then will open the meeting up to staff concerns. One of the concerns is that there are union organizers in the hospital looking for support. The director knows this is a very delicate situation and must be handled carefully due to laws about free speech and assembly.

Exercise 9-19: *Multiple-choice question*
The director is approached by union organizers and the best response is:
    A. Take the information and walk away
    B. Ask them to leave
    C. Call security
    D. Refuse to take the information

After the team meeting, the director answers some of Jacob's questions about managing personnel. At the meeting, Jacob recognizes one of the staff members who was drunk the other night at a local club where Jacob was with some of his

Answers to this chapter begin on page 125.

friends. Without divulging names he asks the director what would be the right thing to do.

Exercise 9-20: *Multiple-choice question*
A staff person was noted drunk in a club on the staff person's day off. The director should:

        A. Refer the staff member to counseling

        B. Ask the staff member about the incident directly

        C. Do nothing

        D. Suspend the staff member for unprofessional behavior

The director says that staff issues come up all the time and she has to use management principles to deal with them logically.

Exercise 9-21: *Multiple-choice question*
A staff member comes into the office and complains about another staff member not completing his or her work. The staff member should be told by the director to:

        A. Finish the work

        B. Talk to the other person first

        C. Document the incident

        D. Come back with the person

The director does tell Jacob there are specific cases that are serious and the chain of command is not encouraged as it is in the usual conflict management cases.

Exercise 9-22: *Select all that apply*
Instances in which a staff member needs to report an occurrence directly to the manager include:

    ❑ A health care professional diverting drugs

    ❑ A conflict between the unlicensed assistive personnel and nurse

    ❑ An unprofessional comment from a physician to a nurse

    ❑ A patient states a nurse made a sexual advance

    ❑ A nurse makes a sexual comment to a pharmacist

    ❑ A patient complains about the care received on the prior shift

As they are talking about staff issues, a staff member comes into the office to report that one of her colleagues is making excessive personal phone calls and the work in the nurse's pod is falling behind. The director asks the staff person to approach the person making the phone calls and inquire if everything is okay because this is out of pattern. The nurse comes back and says that there is a personal problem going on and that the person needs to be in touch with the family.

Answers to this chapter begin on page 125.

Exercise 9-23: *Multiple-choice question*

The best response the director can make to this situation is:

      A. Tell the person making phone calls to go home

      B. Tell the person complaining to stop complaining

      C. Tell the person making phone calls to use her private office phone

      D. Tell the person complaining to pick up the other person's assignment

Just then a call comes in from the triage area. The patient load has just increased tremendously due to a multi-vehicle accident. The director calls the supervisor to see if they can send help.

Exercise 9-24: *Multiple-choice question*

The supervisor "pulls" a staff member from the ICU where three patients have been discharged and tells the staff member to report to the ED triage unit. The staff member states that she is not comfortable triaging. The best response by the supervisor is:

      A. "Go or you will get fired for insubordination."

      B. "I understand your feeling but you need to go."

      C. "I understand your feelings but they are not the issue."

      D. "You don't have to go if you can find me someone who will."

Jacob asks under what situations do you consider abandonment of patient care by a nurse.

Exercise 9-25: *Select all that apply*

A nurse is considered to have abandoned patients when:

    ❑ A nurse gets a call to take another admission and says this is ridiculous and leaves the unit

    ❑ A nurse gets a call to take another admission and says this is ridiculous and calls the supervisor to refuse

    ❑ A nurse leaves the building grounds for a cigarette because it is a no-smoking campus

    ❑ A nurse refuses to come in for overtime when the unit is busy

    ❑ A nurse refuses to stay when the unit is busy

    ❑ A nurse refuses to stay in a state of emergency

As they are speaking, a staff member, visibly upset, comes in and says a suspicious package has been found in the waiting room.

Answers to this chapter begin on page 125.

Exercise 9-26: *Multiple-choice question*

Upon finding a brown paper-wrapped package in the ED on the floor next to the elevator, the staff nurse should:

     A. Call 911

     B. Open the package to see what is inside

     C. Call security

     D. Run the package to the parking lot

After that crisis is over, Jacob and the director talk about other staff disciplinary issues. The director tells Jacob that staff are usually given up to three warnings about an incident or unprofessional behavior. So in other words they are warned, they are warned a second time, and if the same or related behavior occurs a third time, they are terminated. But the director tells Jacob that he works very closely with Human Resources (HR) when it comes to employee issues of hiring and firing. Jacob tells the director that he is scheduled to spend a day in the HR department; the director encourages him to write questions down for the HR director.

Jacob has learned a tremendous amount today about patient management, staff management, and the work environment. He has taken many notes to share with his classmates!

Answers to this chapter begin on page 125.

Answers

Exercise 9-1: *Multiple-choice question*
Core measures are outcome data mandated of health care organizations by which agency?
  A. National Patient Safety Goals—NO
  B. The Joint Commission –YES, they are part of TJC's patient safety goals.
  C. Centers for Disease Control and Prevention—NO
  D. Agency for Healthcare Research and Quality—NO

Exercise 9-2: *Select all that apply*
A core measure for pneumonia is measured by the following actions:
☐ Coughing, turning, and deep breathing patients every 2 hours—NO, although this is good practice.
☒ **Providing antibiotics within 4 hours of admission—YES**
☐ Ensuring respiratory therapy is consulted—NO, although this is good practice.
☐ Mouth care—NO, although this is good practice.
☒ **Acting on the information from cultures—YES**
☐ Decreasing suctioning—NO, although this is good practice.

Exercise 9-3: *Multiple-choice question*
The case manager notifies the primary care provider (PCP), who is in surgery, that the patient's insurance will not pay for another day's stay. What should the case manager do?
  A. Call the family to pick up the patient—NO, this does not ensure they are discharged properly.
  B. Notify the nursing supervisor of the situation—NO, the nurse can try to amend the situation.
  C. Ask accounting to change the patient's status to nonpay—NO, this is not feasible.
  D. **Wait for the primary care provider—YES, the PCP must attend to the situation.**

Exercise 9-4: *Multiple-choice question*
A patient has a neck injury and is unable to swallow well. What interdisciplinary intervention should the nurse include in the patient's care plan?
  A. Ask the family to bring protein shakes—NO
  B. Ask the doctor for TPN—NO
  C. **Request a dietitian referral—YES, this is the best intervention.**
  D. Request an occupational therapy referral—NO

Exercise 9-5: *Multiple-choice question*
The nurse on a pediatric unit has a patient for the second time, an 8-year-old girl. The nurse remembers asking the parents to have the child's eyes checked because the child sits so close to the television and the parents have not followed through. The nurse should:
  A. Discuss the importance of eye exams—NO, this has already been done.
  B. Ask the PCP for a referral—NO, this has already been done.
  C. Get a family history of eye disorders—NO, this has already been done.
  D. **Find out if they can afford the care—YES, it may be an access-to-care situation.**

Exercise 9-6: *Multiple-choice question*
An emergency department (ED) nurse takes report on three patients. One patient is a 24-hour observe and it is hour 23. The best action for the nurse would be:
  A. Discharge the patient—NO, this needs an order.
  B. **Call the PCP to discharge the patient—YES**
  C. Transfer the patient to an in-patient unit and status—NO, this needs an order.
  D. Wait to see if the PCP makes round this shift—NO, this is costing the organization money.

Exercise 9-7: *Multiple-choice question*
The nurse is discharging a postpartum patient who has a flat affect and a history of postpartum depression (PPD). Which is the appropriate referral?
  A. Primary care office—NO
  B. PPD support group—NO, she is not ready for a group format initially.
  C. Mother and infant play group—NO, this does not address the problem.
  D. **Mental health counselor—YES**

Exercise 9-8: *Multiple-choice question*
A day-shift nurse complains to the unit director that the night shift never gets their work done and now the day shift is behind. The best response by the unit director is:
  A. "I will talk to them."—NO, this is alleviating the nurse of his or her professional responsibility.
  B. "They usually do their best but must have gotten busy."—NO, this does not solve the issue.
  C. "You should call a group meeting."—NO, this will cause resentment.
  D. **"Provide me with examples of what you mean."—YES, assessment is the first step in any nursing situation.**

Exercise 9-9: *Multiple-choice question*
The lowest percent of patients that needs to be surveyed about satisfaction post discharge for reimbursement is:
  A. **5%—YES**
  B. 10%—NO, although many hospitals survey more than the required amount of patients.

C. 25%—NO, although many hospitals survey more than the required amount of patients.

D. 50%—NO, although many hospitals survey more than the required amount of patients.

Exercise 9-10: *Select all that apply*

The most important information collected on patient satisfaction surveys normally includes the following:

☒ **Accessibility to care—YES, this includes convenient places for care, time waited for care, and cost.**

☒ **Communication skills of all providers—YES, this is probably the most important attribute of all health care situations.**

☒ **Quality of care provided—YES, this is important.**

☒ **Dietary, lab, testing, and valet parking services—YES, these are important to patients.**

❑ Appearance of health care providers—NO, this is not surveyed specifically.

☒ **Facilities' quality—YES, the room and unit are important aspects.**

Exercise 9-11: *Multiple-choice question*

First-level managers are responsible for unit operations:

A. During the day shift while they are there—NO, this is not their complete responsibility.

B. If it pertains to specific issues only on that unit—NO, how their unit interacts with other units is their responsibility.

C. **24/7—YES**

D. When the leader of all critical care units is off—NO, although managers can cover for each other.

Exercise 9-12: *Multiple-choice question*

A 16-year-old is in Bay 4 and has been told she has gonorrhea. She is crying and wants reassurance that no one will find out about this condition. The nurse's best response to the patient is:

A. "You must tell your sexual partners so they can get treated."—NO, this is not the most important response.

B. "You should tell your parents because they are going to see the health care bill."—NO

C. "Due to HIPAA regulations the information will be kept confidential."—NO

D. **"Gonorrhea is a reportable disease to the Public Health Department."—YES, gonorrhea is a reportable disease and the Public Health Department tries to contact the person's partners if possible.**

Exercise 9-13: *Multiple-choice question*

A patient being admitted for worsening dementia and urinary tract infection is wandering in the hall and states, "I am looking for the 5 and 10 cent store to buy a candy bar." The nurse's best response is:

A. "I will show you where the store is" and leads the patient back to his bay.—NO, do not play into the delusion.

B. "This is the ED of a hospital not the 5 and 10 cent store."—NO, this is not helpful in getting the patient to safety.

C. "Let's talk about why you need to go to the store."—NO, this is not helpful in getting the patient to safety.

D. **"Let me help you back to your bed."—YES, this redirects them to reality.**

Exercise 9-14: *Multiple-choice question*

The best nursing intervention for this patient with dementia would be:

A. Restrain him—NO, this is always the last resort.

B. **Place him in a bay close to the nurses' station—YES, this will help everyone keep an eye on him.**

C. Call the family to sit with him—NO, this may not be feasible but if it is, it is a good idea for some parts of the day.

D. Call the supervisor to get him on a locked unit—NO, this is not the first response because this will depend on bed availability.

Exercise 9-15: *Multiple-choice question*

The patient in Bay 10 is diaphoretic and on the floor. He is ashen in color and states he just passed out but doesn't know why and feels like he has pain in his arm. The first thing the nurse should do is:

A. **Call the rapid response team—YES, do not waste time; summon help!**

B. Give him oxygen—NO, initially call for help, then apply oxygen.

C. Get him back on the stretcher—NO, this is wasting time too.

D. Get an electrocardiogram—NO

Exercise 9-16: *Multiple-choice question*

A patient's is brought in to the ED and his friends are intoxicated. What should the nurse do?

A. Call 911—NO, this is not a public emergency.

B. Call the local police—NO, this is not a criminal act.

C. Tell them to leave—NO, this may entice them to drive away drunk.

D. **Call security—YES, let them sort it out.**

Exercise 9-17: *Multiple-choice question*

A democratic director would most likely adhere to:

A. Block scheduling that is consistent for each schedule—NO, this does not show flexibility.

B. **Staff self-scheduling—YES, this is decentralized and shows that the leader can relinquish authority to staff.**

C. Centralized scheduling—NO, this does not show flexibility.

D. Taking scheduling requests and trying to honor them—NO, this does not give the staff accountability.

Exercise 9-18: *Select all that apply*

Advantages to working per diem instead of full time are:

☐ Consistent hours—NO, usually there are not set hours.

☐ Lack of health benefits—NO, this is a disadvantage.

☒ **Flexible scheduling—YES, this works well for per-diem nurses.**

☐ Most complex patient load—NO, this should not be the case.

☐ Paid vacation time—NO, this is a disadvantage.

☐ Not working major holidays—NO, many times they must work at least one major holiday.

Exercise 9-19: *Multiple-choice question*

The director is approached by union organizers and the best response is:

A. Take the information and walk away—NO, do not take the information because the director is management.

B. Ask them to leave—NO, this is not the director's call.

C. Call security—NO, this is not the director's call.

D. **Refuse to take the information—YES**

Exercise 9-20: *Multiple-choice question*

A staff person was noted drunk in a club on the staff person's day off. The director should:

A. Refer the staff member to counseling—NO, this is not the responsibility of the director if it does not involve work.

B. Ask the staff member about the incident directly—NO, this is not the responsibility of the director if it does not involve work.

C. **Do nothing—YES, it does not involve work.**

D. Suspend the staff member for unprofessional behavior—NO, this does not involve work.

Exercise 9-21: *Multiple-choice question*
A staff member comes into the office and complains about another staff member not completing his or her work. The staff member should be told by the director to:
  A. Finish the work—NO, this is not the complaining staff member's responsibility.
  B. **Talk to the other person first—YES, follow the chain of command and talk to the person first.**
  C. Document the incident—NO, this is done if there is no resolution.
  D. Come back with the person—NO, this is done if there is no resolution.

Exercise 9-22: *Select all that apply*
Instances in which a staff member needs to report an occurrence directly to the manager include:
☒ **A health care professional diverting drugs—YES, this is a reportable issue and endangers the safety of patients.**
☐ A conflict between the unlicensed assistive personnel and nurse—NO, this can be handled at an individual level.
☐ An unprofessional comment from a physician to a nurse—NO, this can be handled at an individual level.
☒ **A patient states a nurse made a sexual advance—YES, this is a reportable issue and endangers the safety of patients.**
☒ **A nurse makes a sexual comment to a pharmacist—YES, sexual harassment is not tolerated.**
☒ **A patient complains about the care received on the prior shift—YES, patient complaints should be reported so the unit director is aware and can do damage control.**

Exercise 9-23: *Multiple-choice question*
The best response the director can make to this situation is:
  A. Tell the person making phone calls to go home—NO, this is punitive.
  B. Tell the person complaining to stop complaining—NO, this does not address the situation.
  C. **Tell the person making phone calls to use her private office phone—YES, this will be less disruptive to the unit.**
  D. Tell the person complaining to pick up the other person's assignment—NO, this is not that person's responsibility.

Exercise 9-24: *Multiple-choice question*

The supervisor "pulls" a staff member from the ICU where three patients have been discharged and tells the staff member to report to the ED triage unit. The staff member states that she is not comfortable triaging. The best response by the supervisor is:

A. "Go or you will get fired for insubordination."—NO, this is creating conflict.

B. **"I understand your feeling but you need to go."—YES, this is acknowledging feelings without dismissing the responsibility.**

C. "I understand your feelings but they are not the issue."—NO, this is devaluing.

D. "You don't have to go if you can find me someone who will."—NO, this is not the mandate.

Exercise 9-25: *Select all that apply*

A nurse is considered to have abandoned patients when:

☒ **A nurse gets a call to take another admission and says this is ridiculous and leaves the unit—YES, leaving the unit without reporting off to someone is abandonment.**

❑ A nurse gets a call to take another admission and says this is ridiculous and calls the supervisor to refuse—NO, the nurse has not left the unit.

❑ A nurse leaves the building grounds for a cigarette because it is a no-smoking campus—NO, the nurse does not leave the unit for good, just a break.

❑ A nurse refuses to come in for overtime when the unit is busy—NO, this cannot be mandatory.

❑ A nurse refuses to stay when the unit is busy—NO, this cannot be mandatory.

☒ **A nurse refuses to stay in a state of emergency—YES, this is mandatory.**

Exercise 9-26: *Multiple-choice question*

Upon finding a brown paper-wrapped package in the ED on the floor next to the elevator, the staff nurse should:

A. Call 911—NO, this is not the responsibility of the nurse.

B. Open the package to see what is inside—NO, this is not the responsibility of the nurse.

C. **Call security—YES**

D. Run the package to the parking lot—NO, this may trigger an explosive if it is one.

10

Prioritization

Unfolding Case Study #10 ▦ Beyonce

Beyonce is going to leadership clinical today to follow a team leader to understand prioritization of patient care needs. She meets the team leader in the morning and they go over the assignment for today. There is an experienced RN, LPN, and unlicensed assistive personnel on the team for six adult medical patients.

The night shift nurse gives a report on the following six patients:

1. A 52-year-old woman with acute glomerulonephritis
2. A 68-year-old male with hepatitis and liver cirrhosis and esophageal varices
3. A 24-year-old hemophiliac
4. A 60-year-old man with a deep vein thrombosis (DVT) in the left leg
5. A 44-year-old woman who had a left mastectomy yesterday
6. A 72-year-old woman with acute diverticulitis

Exercise 10-1: *Multiple-choice question*
After hearing the morning report, who should Beyonce assess first?

      A. The woman with brown-colored urine who has glomerulonephritis

      B. The man with liver cirrhosis who's complaining of abdominal discomfort

      C. The man with hemophilia who has bleeding into his right elbow joint

      D. The 44-year-old woman with 30 mL of drainage in her Jackson Pratt who had a left mastectomy yesterday

Next, Beyonce and her preceptor check patient laboratory reports.

Exercise 10-2: *Multiple-choice question*
Which report needs to be called to the primary care provider (PCP) first?

      A. The white blood cell count, which is 7.8 mm^3, on the woman who had the mastectomy

      B. The man with cirrhosis who has a cholesterol of 240 mg/dL

    C. The 60-year-old man with a DVT with an international normalized ratio (INR) of 2.5
    D. The woman with glomerulonephritis with a calcium of 7.9 mg/dL

After checking labs, Beyonce checks PCP orders.

Exercise 10-3: *Multiple-choice question*

Which order should the nurse question for the patient with esophageal varices?

    A. Insert a nasogastric tube
    B. Start intravenous D5W at 200 mL/hr
    C. Nothing by mouth (NPO)
    D. Keep head of bed (HOB) in a 30-degree angle

Beyonce asks the preceptor how she will know which patient is the priority. The preceptor tells her there are some guiding principles to go on, but you can never say "always" in nursing because it is a human service. When dealing with humans there are always multiple variables. It takes critical thinking to look at the variables and make a clinical decision. One guideline is Maslow's hierarchy of needs.

Exercise 10-4: *Ordering*

Order the following Maslow hierarchy of needs from 1 to 5:

    _____ Safety
    _____ Esteem
    _____ Physiological
    _____ Self-actualization
    _____ Love and belongingness

Another guideline that Beyonce's preceptor tells her about is physiological before psychological, and the preceptor tells Beyonce of a situation that she has experienced on a surgical unit.

Exercise 10-5: *Multiple-choice question*

On a surgical unit, which patient should the nurse assess first?

    A. A patient with a laparoscopic tubal ligation who is complaining of gastric distension
    B. A patient with a cholecystectomy who is 3 hours postoperative but has not voided
    C. A patient scheduled for a mastectomy who is crying
    D. A patient who has a microscopic prostectomy and is ready to go home

Beyonce's preceptor tells her it is helpful to think of a decision in these terms:

  1. Is it an emergency and if it is, did you summon help?
  2. Is there a safety issue that can be averted?

Answers to this chapter begin on page 137.

3. Are Maslow's hierarchy of needs met?

4. Are the physiological issues more important here than the psychological issues?

5. Most importantly: Do I have enough information or do I need to further assess?

Beyonce understands that prioritizing is about knowing the pathophysiology of conditions as well as being flexible so you allow yourself to make a good clinical decision instead of going through work in a rote manner.

 eResource 10-1: Beyonce recalls a lecture she had in her adult medical-surgical course on the topic of *prioritization*: http://goo.gl/3mjWU

The preceptor provides Beyonce with five clinical situation questions that have come up in the preceptor's past obstetrical experience.

Exercise 10-6: *Multiple-choice question*
While working on a postpartum unit the preceptor was faced with deciding which patient to see first. The preceptor asks Beyonce whom she would see first:

    A. A patient who delivered 4 hours ago and has not voided yet

    B. A patient who is crying because of sore nipples from breastfeeding

    C. A patient who has soaked a Peri-Pad in 3 hours

    D. A patient who is complaining of severe vaginal discomfort

The preceptor now gives Beyonce a newborn nursery scenario.

Exercise 10-7: *Multiple-choice question*
Which infant would the nurse assess first?

    A. A 2-day-old who is visibly jaundiced

    B. A 2-day-old who has voided twice today

    C. A 1-day-old with a heart rate of 180

    D. A 1-day-old who will not breastfeed

Exercise 10-8: *Multiple-choice question*
The triage nursery nurse receives the following phone calls. Which parent should the nurse call back first?

    A. The parent who tells the nurse her 5-month-old cried all night and pulled on her ear

    B. The parent who states that her 2-month-old baby has not had a bowel movement in 24 hours

    C. The parent who reports that her 6-week-old baby is breastfeeding all the time

    D. The parent who states that her 6-week-old vomits after each feeding and is taking long naps

Answers to this chapter begin on page 137.

Exercise 10-9: *Multiple-choice question*
While working in the antepartum clinic, the nurse should assess which patient first?

    A. The woman who is 14 weeks gestation with cheesy white vaginal discharge who is extremely uncomfortable from the itching and irritation

    B. The woman who is 28 weeks gestation with a 9-pound weight gain in 1 week

    C. The women who is 40 weeks gestation who is complaining of urinary incontinence

    D. The woman who is 36 weeks gestation with a white blood cell count of 9.6 mm^3

Just as Beyonce and her preceptor are discussing the obstetrical situations that called for clinical decision making, several call bells go off.

Exercise 10-10: *Multiple-choice question*
Which patient should the most experienced nurse see first?

    A. A 24-year-old hemophiliac who is waiting for discharge instructions

    B. A 60-year-old man with a deep vein thrombosis (DVT) in the left leg who is complaining of shortness of breath

    C. A 44-year-old woman who had a left mastectomy yesterday who has a hematocrit postoperative of 30.2

    D. A 72-year-old woman with acute diverticulitis who is complaining of bloating and gas

Exercise 10-11: *Multiple-choice question*
Later that day a bed opens up in the intensive care unit. Which patient should be transferred to the ICU?

    A. A 68-year-old male with hepatitis and liver cirrhosis and esophageal varices who is bleeding orally

    B. A 24-year-old hemophiliac who is resting comfortably after ice is applied to his elbow

    C. A 44-year-old woman who had a left mastectomy yesterday who has spiked a temperature of 103.1°F

    D. A 72-year-old woman with acute diverticulitis who has not had a bowel movement in 24 hours

Beyonce agrees that prioritizing is difficult and it takes her time to think through each patient's needs and use her decision tree to see if she has enough information to intervene or if further assessment is warranted. Her preceptor does tell her that with experience and practice it gets easier, but that even after 20 years of experience, she needs to stop and think about which patient condition warrants the first response.

Answers to this chapter begin on page 137.

Answers

Exercise 10-1: *Multiple-choice question*

After hearing the morning report, who should Beyonce assess first?

A. The woman with brown-colored urine who has glomerulonephritis—NO, this is a manifestation of the condition.

B. The man with liver cirrhosis who's complaining of abdominal discomfort—NO, this is a manifestation of the condition.

C. **The man with hemophilia who has bleeding into his right elbow joint—YES, the bleeding is active.**

D. The 44-year-old woman with 30 mL of drainage in her Jackson Pratt who had a left mastectomy yesterday—NO, this is within normal limits (WNL).

Exercise 10-2: *Multiple-choice question*

Which report needs to be called to the primary care provider (PCP) first?

A. The white blood cell count, which is 7.8 mm³, on the woman who had the mastectomy—NO, this is WNL.

B. The man with cirrhosis who has a cholesterol of 240 mg/dL—NO, this is high but not life threatening.

C. The 60-year-old man with a DVT with an international normalized ratio (INR) of 2.5—NO, this is normal for someone being treated for a DVT.

D. **The woman with glomerulonephritis with a calcium of 7.9 mg/dL—YES, this is low.**

Exercise 10-3: *Multiple-choice question*

Which order should the nurse question for the patient with esophageal varices?

A. **Insert a nasogastric tube—YES, this could rupture varices.**

B. Start intravenous D5W at 200 mL/hr—NO, this is for hydration.

C. Nothing by mouth (NPO)—NO, this may be appropriate depending on diagnostic testing.

D. Keep head of bed (HOB) in a 30-degree angle—NO, this is appropriate for comfort.

Exercise 10-4: *Ordering*

Order the following Maslow hierarchy of needs from 1 to 5:

__2__ Safety

__3__ Esteem

__1__ Physiological

__5__ Self-actualization

__4__ Love and belongingness

Exercise 10-5: *Multiple-choice question*

On a surgical unit, which patient should the nurse assess first?

A. A patient with a laparoscopic tubal ligation that is complaining of gastric distension—NO, this it not an unexpected complication.

B. A patient with a cholecystectomy who is three hours postoperative but has not voided—NO, this may be due to dehydration.

C. **A patient scheduled for a mastectomy who is crying—YES, the patient is very upset and in this case psychosocial takes precedence over physical.**

D. A patient who has a microscopic prostectomy and is ready to go home—NO, this is not urgent.

Exercise 10-6: *Multiple-choice question*

Working on a post-partum unit the preceptor was faced with deciding which patient to see first. The preceptor asks Beyonce whom she would see first.

A. A patient who delivered 4 hours ago and has not voided yet—NO, this is not urgent.

B. A patient who is crying because of sore nipples from breastfeeding—NO, this is also not urgent.

C. A patient who has soaked a Peri-Pad in 3 hours—NO, this is normal post delivery.

D. **A patient who is complaining of severe vaginal discomfort—YES, this may mean a hematoma.**

Exercise 10-7: *Multiple-choice question*

Which infant would the nurse assess first?

A. A 2-day-old who is visibly jaundice—NO, this is not urgent.

B. A 2-day-old who has voided twice today—NO, this is within normal limits (WNL).

C. **A 1-day-old with a heart rate of 180—YES, a heart rate above 160 is not WNL.**

D. A 1-day-old who will not breastfeed—NO, this is a priority but the tachycardia is more life threatening.

Exercise 10-8: *Multiple-choice question*

The triage nursery nurse receives the following phone calls. Which parent should the nurse call back first?

A. The parent who tells the nurse her 5 month old cried all night and pulled on her ear—NO, this is indicative of an ear infection.

B. The parent who states that her 2-month-old baby has not had a bowel movement in 24 hours—NO, this is not an emergency.

C. The parent who reports that her 6-week-old baby is breastfeeding all the time—NO, this may be a normal growth spurt.

D. **The parent who states her 6-week-old vomits after each feeding and is taking long naps—YES, this may be a condition that leads to dehydration.**

Exercise 10-9: *Multiple-choice question*
While working in the antepartum clinic, the nurse should assess which patient first?

A. The woman who is 14 weeks gestation with cheesy white vaginal discharge who is extremely uncomfortable from the itching and irritation—NO, this is typical signs of a yeast infection.

B. **The woman who is 28 weeks gestation with a 9-pound weight gain in one week—YES, this may indicate that there is edema which may be a symptom of PIH (pregnancy-induced hypertension).**

C. The women who is 40 weeks gestation who is complaining of urinary incontinence—NO, this is typical of an enlarged uterus pressing on the bladder.

D. The woman who is 36 weeks gestation with a WBC count of 9.6 mm³—NO, this is within normal limits (WNL).

Exercise 10-10: *Multiple-choice question*
Which patient should the most experienced nurse see first?

A. A 24-year-old hemophiliac who is waiting for discharge instructions—NO, this is not urgent.

B. **A 60-year-old man with a deep vein thrombosis (DVT) in the left leg who is complaining of shortness of breath—YES, this may indicate a pulmonary emboli.**

C. A 44-year-old woman who had a left mastectomy yesterday who has a hematocrit postoperative of 30.2—NO, this is low but not urgent.

D. A 72-year-old woman with acute diverticulitis who is complaining of bloating and gas—NO, these are symptoms of the condition.

Exercise 10-11: *Multiple-choice question*
Later that day a bed opens up in the ICU, which patient should be transferred to the ICU?

A. **A 68-year-old male with hepatitis and liver cirrhosis and esophageal varices who is bleeding orally—YES, the potential for hemorrhage is great.**

B. A 24-year-old hemophiliac who is resting comfortably after ice is applied to his elbow—NO, this is not critical.

C. A 44-year-old woman who had a left mastectomy yesterday who has spiked a temperature of 103.1°F—NO, this is not critical.

D. A 72-year-old woman with acute diverticulitis who has not had a bowel movement in 24 hours—NO, this is not critical.

11

Health Care Finances

Unfolding Case Study #11 ▪ Jacob

Jacob is spending the day with the financial manager of the health care organization in order to fulfill his leadership clinical requirement to understand the fiscal responsibility of an RN.

Exercise 11-1: *Select all that apply*

Correct budgeting is important for:

- ❑ Economic stability of the organization
- ❑ Manager bonuses for incentives
- ❑ Decreasing escalating health care costs
- ❑ Providing safe and effective care
- ❑ Increasing insurance reimbursement margins
- ❑ Decreasing health care mistakes

Jacob's preceptor meets him and tells him that they are going to discuss finances all day and actually go to a unit budget meeting. The preceptor explains to Jacob that the fiscal year for the hospital is from July 1 to June 30 in any given year.

 eResource 11-1: As a review, the preceptor asks Jacob what he knows about *Financial Statements: What Are They? What Do They Mean?* http://goo.gl/IkJg3

Exercise 11-2: *Multiple-choice question*

The largest part of a health care budget is paid to:

- A. Physicians
- B. Nurses
- C. Administration
- D. Support staff

Answers to this chapter begin on page 147.

Exercise 11-3: *Multiple-choice question*

The largest portion of health care expenditure goes to:

    A. New facilities

    B. Diagnostic machinery

    C. Patient care supplies

    D. Patient care delivery

The unit point-of-care budget meeting is first thing in the morning. The nurse manager provides staff with the unit's budget report. One of the staff nurses asks why supply costs are so high.

Exercise 11-4: *Multiple-choice question*

One of the major ways that supply costs can be decreased on a unit is:

    A. Reuse disposable items after disinfecting

    B. Try to use fewer items on each patient

    C. Change linens only twice a week

    D. Decrease pilfering

Most items from the stock carts are scanned so that they can be replaced. Each item is not charged to a patient's bill but it becomes part of a lump sum received from reimbursement for that diagnostic-related group (DRG). Therefore, if a patient uses fewer supplies, the DRG reimbursement will be more than for the patient who uses more supplies. Personnel budgets are also a big consideration for nurse managers. In the past, hospitals were paid fee-for-service so all services received were paid for, but this is no longer the case.

Exercise 11-5: *Calculation*

If a 1.0 full-time equivalency (FTE) position is based on 40 hours/per week, how many hours does a part-time RN work at a 0.6 level? _____

Exercise 11-6: *Multiple-choice question*

A disadvantage of working part time (PT) or per diem is:

    A. Inconsistent scheduling

    B. Completing competencies

    C. Benefits

    D. Hourly wage

FTE benefits are costly for the organization and are usually calculated at 30% to 40% of the wages.

Exercise 11-7: *Calculation*

If a nurse is making $68,000 a year, what would the nurse's benefits cost the health care organization at a rate of 37%? _____

Answers to this chapter begin on page 147.

The cost of hiring a new nurse is tremendous to the organization. Orientation is extended for nurses, sometimes for a couple of months. Orientation with a preceptor is not calculated into unit work hours.

Exercise 11-8: *Multiple-choice question*
One of the best methods for decreasing orientation costs is:

    A. Decrease orientation time
    B. Use the same preceptor for two new hires
    C. Select candidates carefully
    D. Use computer tutorials and simulation

Unit schedules are made on 4-, 6-, or 8-week cycles. Many units use 12-hour shifts but some use 8-hour shifts while others use a combination. Placing the right mix of staff on a unit is important for safety and to ensure a positive work environment. Some states such as California regulate patient care load to improve safety. Patients admitted to health care organizations have increasing acuity.

Exercise 11-9: *Multiple-choice question*
All items and personnel for one unit are stated to be derived from a single:

    A. Cost center
    B. Capital budget
    C. Operation budget
    D. Revenue budget

The preceptor tells Jacob that health care costs are a national issue as is access to health care. The preceptor explains that the intent of health care reform is to address these concerns.

 eResource 11-2: Jacob remembers learning about the history of health care reform in the United States, visiting the Kaiser Family Foundation website: http://goo.gl/8YTF3

Exercise 11-10: *Select all that apply*
Lack of health care access includes the following factors:

    ❑ Lack of specialists
    ❑ Uninsured or underinsured individuals
    ❑ Cultural disparity
    ❑ Prescription drug costs
    ❑ Transportation
    ❑ Increase in outpatient facilities

The preceptor explains that health care is paid for by the government, private insurance companies, and individuals. Uninsured patients raise everyone's cost. Insurance has been around for over 100 years.

Answers to this chapter begin on page 147.

Exercise 11-11: *Matching*

Match the type of insurance in Column A to the description of payment in Column B.

Column A	Column B
A. Health maintenance organization (HMO)	_____ A group of providers and organizations take care of patients usually with co-pay
B. Preferred provider organization (PPO)	_____ Managed care for a geographical area
C. Point-of-service (POS) organization	_____ Must choose a provider in network
D. Medicare	_____ Long-term care for those with poor income
E. Medicaid	_____ Government insurance for individuals 65 and older

> **eResource 11-3:** Jacob remembers reading about health care costs online: [Pathway: www.kaiseredu.org → select "Cost and Spending" and "U.S. Health Care Costs" to review key content]

The preceptor explains to Jacob that patients have other concerns about hospital bills including prescription drug costs.

Exercise 11-12: *Multiple-choice question*

The Medicare part that provides coverage for patients to purchase prescription medication is:

    A. Part A
    B. Part B
    C. Part C
    D. Part D

Another service Medicare pays for is hospice services, which include respite services. Jacob asks what respite services are and the preceptor tells him they are services provided to families caring for a terminally ill member so the family can get away for a while and have the patient cared for.

Exercise 11-13: *Multiple-choice question*

Medicare provides for hospice services for what length of time?

    A. 90 days
    B. 6 months
    C. 1 year
    D. As long as needed

> **eResource 11-4:** For an overview of the health care benefits that pay for hospice, Jacob views *Paying for Hospice Care:* http://goo.gl/xRj1T

Answers to this chapter begin on page 147.

The preceptor tells Jacob that there are different levels of care that are paid for also. The trend is to increase incentive for primary care rather than spending most of U.S. health care dollars on tertiary care.

Exercise 11-14: *Multiple-choice question*
At a health fair the nurse is performing cholesterol screenings. This is an example of:

    A. Primary care
    B. Secondary care
    C. Tertiary care
    D. Triaging

Exercise 11-15: *Multiple-choice question*
A patient is placed in rehabilitation after a hip replacement. This is an example of:

    A. Primary care
    B. Secondary care
    C. Tertiary care
    D. Triaging

Exercise 11-16: *Multiple-choice question*
The school nurse is examining a child in grade school and sends him to the emergency department (ED) because of suspected appendicitis. This is an example of:

    A. Primary care
    B. Secondary care
    C. Tertiary care
    D. Triaging

 eResource 11-5: Jacob reinforces his understanding of the levels of prevention by playing the *Levels of Prevention* game on Wisc-Online: http://goo.gl/sZbLd

The preceptor also tells Jacob about the increasing importance of veterans care. The Veterans Health Administration is a system set up to provide health care services to veterans and their families. There is a great concern currently for veterans coming home with head injuries related to sniper bombings and posttraumatic stress disorder. This is a major concern for health care providers and will be an increasing concern in the future.

Jacob is amazed that he learned so much today about health care finances with his preceptor. The most significant thing that he has learned is how responsible nurses, as front-line providers, are for financial considerations.

Answers to this chapter begin on page 147.

Answers

Exercise 11-1: *Select all that apply*

Correct budgeting is important for:

☒ **Economic stability of the organization—YES, this ensures accessibility and jobs.**

☐ Manager bonuses for incentives—NO, this is not an important reason to monitor health care costs.

☒ **Decreasing escalating health care costs—YES, this is important for our nation.**

☒ **Providing safe and effective care—YES, saving money will ensure that more people can receive care.**

☒ **Increasing insurance reimbursement margins—YES, this assists the hospital to become solvent.**

☒ **Decreasing health care mistakes—YES, this has to do with being an efficient organization.**

Exercise 11-2: *Multiple-choice question*

The largest part of a health care budget is paid to:

A. Physicians—NO

B. **Nurses—YES, nursing is the largest cost because of the numbers needed.**

C. Administration—NO

D. Support staff—NO

Exercise 11-3: *Multiple-choice question*

The largest portion of health care expenditure goes to:

A. New facilities—NO

B. Diagnostic machinery—NO

C. Patient care supplies—NO

D. **Patient care delivery—YES, it is personnel costs.**

Exercise 11-4: *Multiple-choice question*
One of the major ways that supply costs can be decreased on a unit is:
  A. Reuse disposable items after disinfecting—NO, this breaks down the disposable plastic and makes it unsafe.
  B. Try to use fewer items on each patient—NO, although this helps it is not the major culprit.
  C. Change linens only twice a week—NO, most organizations do it every other day.
  D. **Decrease pilfering—YES, this is a tremendous hospital cost.**

Exercise 11-5: *Calculation*
If a 1.0 full-time equivalency (FTE) position is based on 40 hours/per week, how many hours does a part-time RN work at a 0.6 level? **24 hours per week**

Exercise 11-6: *Multiple-choice question*
A disadvantage of working part time (PT) or per diem is:
  A. Inconsistent scheduling—NO, this is an advantage for many.
  B. Completing competencies—NO, this has to be done by all nurses.
  C. **Benefits—YES, these are usually not paid.**
  D. Hourly wage—NO, this may in some cases be higher than full-timers.

Exercise 11-7: *Calculation*
If a nurse is making $68,000 a year, what would the nurse's benefits cost the health care organization at a rate of 37%? **$25,160**

Exercise 11-8: *Multiple-choice question*
One of the best methods for decreasing orientation costs is:
  A. Decrease orientation time—NO, this may produce an unsafe situation.
  B. Use the same preceptor for two new hires—NO, this does not accomplish the individualized guidance needed.
  C. **Select candidates carefully—YES, decreased turnover is the best method.**
  D. Use computer tutorials and simulation—NO, this does not replace hands-on orientation.

Exercise 11-9: *Multiple-choice question*
All items and personnel for one unit are stated to be derived from a single:
  A. **Cost center—YES, each unit has its own cost center to maintain control of their budget.**
  B. Capital budget—NO, this is for large item purchases.
  C. Operation budget—NO, this is the budget need to run the unit day to day.
  D. Revenue budget—NO, this is the money made.

Exercise 11-10: *Select all that apply*

Lack of health care access includes the following factors:

☐ Lack of specialists—NO, there are plenty of specialists but a lack of primary care providers.

☒ **Uninsured or underinsured individuals—YES, people with no insurance seek health care less often.**

☒ **Cultural disparity—YES, people of different cultures are marginalized in the U.S. system.**

☒ **Prescription drug costs—YES, these are expensive for many.**

☒ **Transportation—YES, this may be an issue.**

☐ Increase in outpatient facilities—NO, this should assist with access.

Exercise 11-11: *Matching*

Match the type of insurance in Column A to the description of payment in Column B.

Column A	Column B
A. Health maintenance organization (HMO)	__B__ A group of providers and organizations take care of patients usually with co-pay
B. Preferred provider organization (PPO)	__A__ Managed care for a geographical area
C. Point-of-service (POS) organization	__C__ Must choose a provider in network
D. Medicare	__E__ Long-term care for those with poor income
E. Medicaid	__D__ Government insurance for individuals 65 and older

Exercise 11-12: *Multiple-choice question*

The Medicare part that provides coverage for patients to purchase prescription medication is:

A. Part A—NO, this is hospital insurance.

B. Part B—NO, this is for outpatient services.

C. Part C—NO, this is for supplemental insurance purchase.

D. **Part D—YES, prescriptions are available to those with part D.**

Exercise 11-13: *Multiple-choice question*

Medicare provides for hospice services for what length of time?

A. 90 days—NO

B. 6 months—NO, the patient has to be expected to die within 6 months but if he or she does not, hospice can be extended.

C. One year—NO

D. **As long as needed—YES, the patient can be recertified every 90 days when terminally ill.**

Exercise 11-14: *Multiple-choice question*

At a health fair the nurse is performing cholesterol screenings. This is an example of:

  A. Primary care—NO, this is decreasing risks.

  B. **Secondary care—YES, this is prevention and early intervention.**

  C. Tertiary care—NO, this is treatment.

  D. Triaging—NO, this is emergency and disaster management.

Exercise 11-15:

A patient is placed in rehabilitation after a hip replacement. This is an example of:

  A. Primary care—NO, this is decreasing risks.

  B. Secondary care—NO, this is prevention and early intervention.

  C. **Tertiary care—YES, this is treatment.**

  D. Triaging—NO, this is emergency and disaster management.

Exercise 11-16: *Multiple-choice question*

The school nurse is examining a child in grade school and sends him to the emergency department (ED) because of a suspected appendicitis. This is an example of:

  A. Primary care—NO, this is decreasing risks.

  B. **Secondary care—YES, this is prevention and early intervention.**

  C. Tertiary care—NO, this is treatment.

  D. Triaging—NO, this is emergency and disaster management.

12

Legal Issues

Unfolding Case Study #12 ▨ Roxanne

The next class concerns legal issues that every nurse needs to know. Dr. Bennett tells the class that from day 1 in clinical practice they need to practice defensively. Yes! He tells them this is a society that is legal conscious and humans are human and do make mistakes. The best advice is to follow protocol, assess, and critically think. He reviews some of the basic legal principles and definitions with the class.

Exercise 12-1: *Multiple-choice question*
A nurse should know the nursing regulations of:

      A. The state in which his or her license was obtained

      B. The state in which care is delivered

      C. All in a multicompact state agreement

      D. National standards

Dr. Bennett tells the learners that an organization is obligated to inform the state board of nursing of any disciplinary actions that may occur involving a nurse. Many states have penalties for not informing the board of nursing in a timely manner.

Exercise 12-2: *Select all that apply*
A state board of nursing sanction can arise from the following situations:

      ❑ Impaired nursing practice

      ❑ Negligence

      ❑ Incompetence

      ❑ Medication error resulting in harm

      ❑ Abuse

      ❑ Fraud

      ❑ Practicing outside the scope of nursing

Answers to this chapter begin on page 159.

eResource 12-1: To reinforce the students' understanding of the nurse's responsibility regarding an impaired nurse, Dr. Bennett has the class read an article, "The Impaired Nurse: Would You Know What to Do if You Suspected Substance Abuse?": http://goo.gl/ZhAEc

Exercise 12-3: *Multiple-choice question*
Of the following actions, which one is reportable to the state board of nursing?
- A. A nurse leaves in the middle of the shift without notification
- B. A nurse who befriends a patient on Facebook after the patient is discharged
- C. A nurse who receives a driving under the influence (DUI)
- D. A nurse who makes a medication error that causes a patient to code

Exercise 12-4: *Multiple-choice question*
Of the following actions, which one is reportable to the state board of nursing?
- A. A nurse receives a report from an unlicensed assistive personnel (UAP) that the patient is short of breath and does not assess the patient and the patient codes
- B. A nurse makes a medication error and the patient has an allergic reaction
- C. A nurse hangs the wrong blood but recognizes it before the patient reacts
- D. A nurse is verbally abusive to a coworker

Dr. Bennett tells the class that the health care organization has responsibilities to the employees, as well as the employees having responsibility to the patients and public.

Exercise 12-5: *Select all that apply*
The health care organization is responsible to:
- ❑ Hire, maintain, and supervise qualified and competent staff
- ❑ Ensure practitioners maintain private malpractice insurance
- ❑ Maintain equipment in working order
- ❑ Maintain areas for staff to eat and get away from work for breaks
- ❑ Maintain a civil atmosphere for employees
- ❑ Maintain a safe physical environment

Next, Dr. Bennett ensures that the learners understand legal terms that are often used when speaking about patient incidences.

Answers to this chapter begin on page 159.

Exercise 12-6: *Matching*

Match the term in Column A to its description in Column B.

Column A	Column B
A. Malpractice	_____ Discussing or displaying private patient information publicly
B. Tort Law	_____ Care a reasonable nurse would deliver
C. Negligence	_____ Wrongful physical contact with a patient
D. Standard of care	_____ A private or civil wrong
E. Breach of confidentiality	_____ Producing fear or apprehension in a patient
F. Defamation of character	_____ Failure to act in a reasonably prudent manner
G. Assault	_____ Restraining a patient against his or her will
H. Battery	_____ Telling untruths or damaging information about a patient
I. False imprisonment	_____ Failure to safeguard a patient

Dr. Bennett goes into a bit more detail about malpractice because that is an area all health professionals are most concerned about. Malpractice is sometimes called *professional negligence* and is *nonintentional*. For a malpractice suit to be successful there must be six elements.

Exercise 12-7: *Matching*

Match the element of malpractice in Column A to its description in Column B.

Column A	Column B
A. Duty	_____ Actions or lack of actions by the nurse caused harm
B. Breach of duty	_____ Patient sustained a condition of physical harm
C. Foreseeability	_____ Patient is owed a specific level of care
D. Causation	_____ Additional nonfunctioning time or damages were incurred by the patient
E. Injury	_____ Failure to provide standard of care
F. Damages	_____ Events can be expected

Dr. Bennett breaks the class into small groups to work on a malpractice case and identify the components. They were given the Lewis Blackman case of the "15-year-old boy who didn't have to die" (http://www.lewisblackman.net).

Lewis was admitted to a health care facility for an elective surgery and was given Toradol for postoperative pain. The pain medication produced ulcerations in his gastrointestinal tract and he eventually died from an internal hemorrhage. This tragic case unfolds over several days.

Answers to this chapter begin on page 159.

Roxanne, Beyonce, and Jacob review the case and identify the elements of malpractice and report their case findings to the class.

Exercise 12-8: *Matching*

Match the element of malpractice in Column A to its description of the Lewis Blackman case in Column B.

Column A	Column B
A. Duty	_____ By not ordering a complete blood count, the hemorrhage went undetected
B. Breach of duty	_____ Patient sustains an internal bleed
C. Foreseeability	_____ Patient is not weighed until the mother insists
D. Causation	_____ Loss of life
E. Injury	_____ Nurse does not assess distended abdomen but tells patient to ambulate
F. Damages	_____ Administers a toxic drug when patient has no output

Roxanne asks a question in class, "Should nurses have their own personal liability insurance?" Dr. Bennett answers absolutely they should.

Exercise 12-9: *Select all that apply*

Nurses should carry their own liability insurance because:

❑ The organization will not cover them

❑ Patients may sue them but sue physicians more

❑ Patients mistrust nursing

❑ Nurses are sued the most

❑ Nurses can get sued separate from the organization

❑ It is mandated by the state boards of nursing

Dr. Bennett provides the class with information about the legal process should they be called to provide a *deposition* or testimony in a case.

Exercise 12-10: *Select all that apply*

A nurse is called by the hospital lawyer because the nurse is named in a suit involving a patient the nurse cared for 11 months ago. When requested to give a deposition, a nurse should:

❑ Describe in detail what happened when asked by the lawyers

❑ Review the chart before the deposition

❑ Schedule it when the nurse gets off work

❑ Use body language effectively in the session

❑ Ask other nurses if they have been called also

❑ Always have your own lawyer present

Answers to this chapter begin on page 159.

The class goes over some lessons on good charting. Documentation, either paper or electronic health record (EHR), should be:

- Easy to read
- Objective
- Accurate
- Complete
- Timely

 eResource 12-2: To help the class better understand their responsibilities, Dr. Bennett:
   - Shows the class a video, *Documentation: Avoiding the Pitfalls*, in which a lawyer discusses the importance of proper documentation: http://youtu.be/yeFr66flhXg
   - Gives the class an article to read: "Nursing Documentation: Let's Get Back to Basics": http://goo.gl/BFtHZ
   - Provides a documentation template: http://goo.gl/kkeHB

Exercise 12-11: *Multiple-choice question*
Which documentation entry does not follow the rules of good charting?
   A. "Ambulated in hall with encouragement."
   B. "Refused to ambulate as encouraged."
   C. "Ambulated in hall for 15 minutes."
   D. "Ambulated after I told the patient of risks of bed rest."

Exercise 12-12: *Multiple-choice question*
Which documentation entry does not follow the rules of good charting?
   A. "Pain medication provided at 0200 for pain rated at 8 out of 10."
   B. "Additional pain medication provided for pain that pt. states would not go away."
   C. "Pt. complains of pain every 2 hours."
   D. "Pain medication outcome rated at 3, 30 minutes after pain medication."

 eResource 12-3: To supplement the class discussion regarding documentation, Dr. Bennett shows the class:
   - South Carolina Department of Health and Human Services' Documentation Guidelines: http://goo.gl/O4F6j
   - A presentation on nursing considerations related to documentation: http://goo.gl/WIzkI

After class Roxanne prepares for the next day in which she will shadow the hospital lawyer and learn more about the intricacies of health care liability. She meets the lawyer the next morning who is also a nurse. The lawyer tells Roxanne that the first task of the day will be to review *incident* or *occurrence reports* made out by nurses in the institution.

Answers to this chapter begin on page 159.

Exercise 12-13: *Multiple-choice question*

The purpose of filling out an incident report is:

       A. To notify risk management of serious incidents

       B. To identify nurses who are at risk for malpractice suits

       C. To identify nursing care units that need further in-services on policies

       D. To notify hospital administration that a problem exists with communication

The lawyer asks Roxanne the following question to stimulate her critical thinking about incidence or occurrence reports.

Exercise 12-14: *Multiple-choice question*

A patient falls but is not hurt. After the nurse gets the patient back to bed safely, the first priority is:

       A. Notify the primary care provider (PCP)

       B. Call the patient's durable power of health care to explain what happened and that everything is okay

       C. Fill out an incident report

       D. Call the nursing supervisor

 eResource 12-4: To supplement Roxanne's understanding, the lawyer shows her the National Center for Patient Safety's (NCPS), recommended fall policy: http://goo.gl/g6eMS

The incident report they are reviewing has to do with a patient being restrained in the emergency department (ED). The restraint had to be placed on the patient to protect the patient from hurting himself.

Exercise 12-15: *Multiple-choice question*

Placing a patient in restraints without the patient's approval may be interpreted as _____ if there is not a reasonable safety risk not to intervene.

       A. Assault

       B. Battery

       C. False imprisonment

       D. Neglect

Roxanne and the lawyer go to the inpatient psychiatric unit and look at the patient's EHR for evidence of justification of placing the patient in restraints.

Exercise 12-16: *Select all that apply*

The Omnibus Budget Reconciliation Act (OBRA) of 1987 provides patient rights to be free from physical and chemical restraints and includes the following stipulations if restraints need to be used:

       ❑ There must be a PCP order for specific time and circumstances

       ❑ There must be a PRN (as needed) order for emergencies

Answers to this chapter begin on page 159.

❑ The nurse must continuously assess the patient

❑ The nurse can place the patient in a locked room if needed

❑ Informed consent must be obtained

❑ If the patient is incoherent, informed consent is not needed

The reason the restraints were placed on the patient is stated in the nurse's notes as "numerous attempts to jump off stretcher over the side rails onto broken ankle." The lawyer describes this as protecting the patient, but the PCP should be called first and the order obtained before the restraints are initiated if at all possible. It may even mean that a staff person stays in attendance until the order is received.

 eResource 12-5: The lawyer gives Roxanne an article that discusses the *Problems Associated With the Use of Physical Restraints*: http://goo.gl/4NM8C

Just as they are reviewing the evidence, the lawyer receives a call from the medical unit. The lawyer and Roxanne go to the medical unit and find the following situation. A patient is refusing treatment and packing to leave the hospital.

Exercise 12-17: *Multiple-choice question*

The nurse's priority for a patient who is refusing treatment and packing to exit the hospital is:

    A. Call the PCP to come and talk to the patient

    B. Explain to the patient what the risks will be if the patient leaves

    C. Call the risk manager to assist

    D. Have the patient sign an Against Medical Advice (AMA) form

 eResource 12-6: To reinforce her understanding of patient's rights, Roxanne consults her mobile device to review information regarding a patient's rights to refuse treatment: http://goo.gl/JkPj8

After the crisis on the medical unit, the lawyer goes over another important issue with Roxanne, *informed consent*. Nurses are frequently called to be witnesses to informed consent. Roxanne asks a great question, "Why are some procedures done without informed consent?" The lawyer explains that the general hospital admission consent is signed by all patients and it stipulates that hospital personnel are able to perform routine procedures and, in the case of an emergency, they can act. Other procedures that are not routine and are invasive need an informed consent.

Exercise 12-18: *Multiple-choice question*

Which of the following procedures would warrant an informed consent?

    A. Starting a peripheral intravenous line

    B. Drawing blood gases on a patient in respiratory distress

    C. Placing a peripherally inserted central catheter (PICC)

    D. Starting a chemotherapeutic agent

Answers to this chapter begin on page 159.

The lawyer further explains to Roxanne that there are three considerations to each informed consent that nurses should be aware of if they are witnessing the consent process with the PCP.

- The patient must have adequate information, including:
  - Diagnosis
  - The purpose of the procedures
  - The risks and benefits of the procedure
  - Alternatives to the procedure
  - Risks and benefits of alternatives to the procedure
  - Risk of declining the procedures
  - The opportunity to ask questions
- The patient must be competent:
  - 18 years of age or older
  - Cognitively able
- Voluntarily

 eResource 12-7: To learn more about informed consent, Roxanne reviews the *ACP Ethics Manual, Sixth Edition*: [Pathway: http://goo.gl/5qvPt → scroll down and select "Informed Decision Making and Consent" and review content]

Exercise 12-19: *Multiple-choice question*

A PCP is obtaining an informed consent from a mother for an infant's circumcision. The mother speaks Spanish and there is a version of the consent form in Spanish. The patient indicates to the nurses and the PCP that she understands by nodding her head when the PCP says the word "circumcision." What is the nurse's responsibility in this situation?

    A. Witness the informed consent

    B. Have a family member who is bilingual verify that the mother understands

    C. Refuse to witness the consent

    D. Obtain a certified interpreter

Roxanne has learned a tremendous amount from her leadership clinical day with the hospital lawyer. She better understands her role in legal situations. She intends to develop a PowerPoint for the rest of her class to present the key issues learned today.

Answers to this chapter begin on page 159.

Answers

Exercise 12-1: *Multiple-choice question*

A nurse should know the nursing regulations of:

 A. The state in which his or her license was obtained—NO, because it may be a multi-state license.

 B. **The state in which care is delivered—YES, a nurse must know the regulations in the state where care is rendered either in person, via the telephone, or web.**

 C. All in a multicompact state agreement—NO, you do not have to know them all.

 D. National standards—NO, there are no national standards; it is regulated state to state.

Exercise 12-2: *Select all that apply*

A state board of nursing sanction can arise from the following situations:

☒ **Impaired nursing practice—YES**

☒ **Negligence—YES**

☒ **Incompetence—YES**

☐ Medication error resulting in harm—NO, it depends if it was individual negligence or a system failure.

☒ **Abuse—YES**

☒ **Fraud—YES**

☒ **Practicing outside the scope of nursing—YES**

Exercise 12-3: *Multiple-choice question*

Of the following actions, which one is reportable to the state board of nursing?

 A. A nurse leaves in the middle of the shift without notification—NO, this is reportable to the manager, then to human resources (HR) for disciplinary action.

 B. A nurse who befriends a patient on Facebook after the patient is discharged—NO, this is not an active nurse-patient relationship.

 C. **A nurse who receives a driving under the influence (DUI)—YES, this is a criminal charge and the board of nursing should be aware.**

 D. A nurse who makes a medication error that causes a patient to code—NO, not unless there was negligence, incompetence, or chemical impairment.

Exercise 12-4: *Multiple-choice question*

Of the following actions, which one is reportable to the state board of nursing?

  A. **A nurse receives a report from a UAP that the patient is short of breath and does not assess the patient and the patient codes—YES, this is neglect.**

  B. A nurse makes a medication error and the patient has an allergic reaction—NO, unless it was negligence or incompetence.

  C. A nurse hangs the wrong blood but recognizes it before the patient reacts—NO, unless it was negligence or incompetence.

  D. A nurse is verbally abusive to a coworker—NO, this is reportable to the manager.

Exercise 12-5: *Select all that apply*

The health care organization is responsible to:

☒ **Hire, maintain, and supervise qualified and competent staff—YES**

❑ Ensure practitioners maintain private malpractice insurance—NO, this is the individuals' responsibility.

☒ **Maintain equipment in working order—YES**

❑ Maintain areas for staff to eat and get away from work for breaks—NO, this is not mandated.

❑ Maintain a civil atmosphere for employees—NO, this is the employees' responsibility.

☒ **Maintain a safe physical environment—YES**

Exercise 12-6: *Matching*

Match the term in Column A to its description in Column B.

Column A	Column B
A. Malpractice	__E__ Discussing or displaying private patient information publicly
B. Tort Law	__D__ Care a reasonable nurse would deliver
C. Negligence	__H__ Wrongful physical contact with a patient
D. Standard of care	__B__ A private or civil wrong
E. Breach of confidentiality	__G__ Producing fear or apprehension in a patient
F. Defamation of character	__A__ Failure to act in a reasonably prudent manner
G. Assault	__I__ Restraining a patient against his or her will
H. Battery	__F__ Telling untruths or damaging information about a patient
I. False imprisonment	__C__ Failure to safeguard a patient

Exercise 12-7: *Matching*

Match the element of malpractice in Column A to its description in Column B.

Column A		Column B
A. Duty	__D__	Actions or lack of actions by the nurse caused harm
B. Breach of duty	__E__	Patient sustained a condition of physical harm
C. Foreseeability	__A__	Patient is owed a specific level of care
D. Causation	__F__	Additional nonfunctioning time or damages were incurred by the patient
E. Injury	__B__	Failure to provide standard of care
F. Damages	__C__	Events can be expected

Exercise 12-8: *Matching*

Match the element of malpractice in Column A to its description of the Lewis Blackman case in Column B.

Column A		Column B
A. Duty	__D__	By not ordering a complete blood count, the hemorrhage went undetected
B. Breach of duty	__E__	Patient sustained an internal bleed
C. Foreseeability	__A__	Patient is not weighed until the mother insists
D. Causation	__F__	Loss of life
E. Injury	__B__	Nurse does not assess distended abdomen but tells patient to ambulate
F. Damages	__C__	Administers a toxic drug when patient has no output

Exercise 12-9: *Select all that apply*

Nurses should carry their own liability insurance because:

❑ The organization will not cover them—NO, they are covered to an extent under the hospital insurance for incidences in which the hospital is sued, not the individual nurse.

❑ Patients may sue them but sue physicians more—NO, this is not always true in today's health care climate.

❑ Patients mistrust nursing—NO, nursing is one of the most trusted professions in the United States.

❑ Nurses are sued the most—NO, hospitals are usually the ones sued.

☒ **Nurses can get sued separate from the organization—YES**

❑ It is mandated by the state boards of nursing—NO, it is not mandated.

Exercise 12-10: *Select all that apply*
A nurse is called by the hospital lawyer because the nurse is named in a suit involving a patient the nurse cared for 11 months ago. When requested to give a deposition, a nurse should:

☐ Describe in detail what happened when asked by the lawyers—NO, just answer the question simply, clearly, and accurately.

☒ **Review the chart before the deposition—YES**

☐ Schedule it when the nurse gets off work—NO, schedule it on a day off when you are not tired.

☐ Use body language effectively in the session—NO, your verbal response needs to be recorded by the court stenographer.

☐ Ask other nurses if they have been called also—NO, do not discuss it with others.

☐ Always have your own lawyer present—NO, this is not always necessary if you are not a primary person named in the case.

Exercise 12-11: *Multiple-choice question*
Which documentation entry does not follow the rules of good charting?
A. "Ambulated in hall with encouragement."—NO, this is factual.
B. "Refused to ambulate as encouraged."—NO, this is factual.
C. "Ambulated in hall for 15 minutes."—NO, this is factual.
D. **"Ambulated after I told the patient of risks of bed rest."—YES, this is subjective; the risks and the teaching done are not specified.**

Exercise 12-12: *Multiple-choice question*
Which documentation entry does not follow the rules of good charting?
A. "Pain medication provided at 0200 for pain rated at 8 out of 10."—NO, this is factual.
B. **"Additional pain medication provided for pain that pt. states would not go away."—YES, this is incomplete; there is no assessment of the pain rating or location.**
C. "Pt. complains of pain every 2 hours."—NO, this is factual.
D. "Pain medication outcome rated at 3, 30 minutes after pain medication."—NO, this is factual.

Exercise 12-13: *Multiple-choice question*
The purpose of filling out an incident report is:
A. **To notify risk management of serious incidents—YES, so trends can be looked at and system issues can be addressed**
B. To identify nurses who are at risk for malpractice suits—NO, this is not the purpose.
C. To identify nursing care units that need further in-services on policies—NO, this is not the purpose because it looks at systems.
D. To notify hospital administration that a problem exists with communication—NO, although communication is the issue in most instances, it can be other things such as timeliness or equipment failure.

Exercise 12-14: *Multiple-choice question*
A patient falls but is not hurt. After the nurse gets the patient back to bed safely, the first priority is:
  A. Notify the primary care provider (PCP)—NO, this can be done after the incident report is completed if the patient is not hurt.
  B. Call the patient's durable power of health care to explain what happened and that everything is okay—NO, this can be done after the incident report is completed if the patient is not hurt.
  C. **Fill out an incident report—YES**
  D. Call the nursing supervisor—NO, this can be done after the incident report is completed if the patient is not hurt because the supervisor will ask the nurse if he or she has filled out the report.

Exercise 12-15: *Multiple-choice question*
Placing a patient in restraints without the patient's approval may be interpreted as _____ if there is not a reasonable safety risk not to intervene.
  A. Assault—NO, this is verbal threats.
  B. Battery—NO, this is physical abuse.
  C. **False imprisonment—YES**
  D. Neglect—NO, this is not doing what a prudent nurse would do in the situation.

Exercise 12-16: *Select all that apply*
The Omnibus Budget Reconciliation Act (OBRA) of 1987 provides patient rights to be free from physical and chemical restraints and includes the following stipulations if restraints need to be used:
☒ **There must be a PCP order for specific time and circumstances—YES**
☐ There must be a PRN order for emergencies—NO, PRN orders are not allowed.
☒ **The nurse must continuously assess the patient—YES, this is done to make sure the patient is safe, does not strangle, or have any skin breakdown.**
☐ The nurse can place the patient in a locked room if needed—NO, this is a restraint.
☒ **Informed consent must be obtained—YES, only in an absolute emergency can it be done without a consent.**
☐ If the patient is incoherent, informed consent is not needed—NO, the durable power of health care needs to be consulted.

Exercise 12-17: *Multiple-choice question*
The nurse's priority for a patient who is refusing treatment and packing to exit the hospital is:
A. Call the PCP to come and talk to the patient—NO, this may be too late.
B. Explain to the patient what the risks will be if they leave—NO, although this is part of the process, it is not the priority.
C. Call the risk manager to assist—NO
D. **Have the patient sign an Against Medical Advice (AMA) form—YES, this tells the person that he or she is taking the responsibility for health care complications.**

Exercise 12-18: *Multiple-choice question*
Which of the following procedures would warrant an informed consent?
A. Starting a peripheral intravenous line—NO, this is considered routine.
B. Drawing blood gases on a patient in respiratory distress—NO, this is considered routine.
C. **Placing a peripherally inserted central catheter (PICC)—YES, this is invasive.**
D. Starting a chemotherapeutic agent—NO, this is considered routine unless the drug is experimental.

Exercise 12-19: *Multiple-choice question*
A PCP is obtaining informed consent from a mother for an infant's circumcision. The mother speaks Spanish and there is a version of the consent form in Spanish. The patient indicates to the nurses and the PCP that she understands by nodding her head when the PCP says the word "circumcision." What is the nurse's responsibility in this situation?
A. Witness the informed consent—NO, the information may not have been understood by the patient.
B. Have a family member who is bilingual verify that the mother understands—NO, the relative may not be familiar with health care terminology.
C. Refuse to witness the consent—NO, this will delay the procedure.
D. **Obtain a certified interpreter—YES, get the language line or an in-house certified interpreter if available.**

13

Human Resources

Unfolding Case Study #13   Beyonce, Jacob, and Roxanne

Beyonce, Jacob, and Roxanne all need to spend a day with the nurse recruiter and human resource (HR) director of a local health care organization because HR is a central office for many internal processes in an organization. HR is responsible not only for hiring and firing, but also for benefits, including worker's compensation insurance, which translates into maintaining a safe environment, and staff competencies in conjunction with the educational department. Another department that HR collaborates with is the central staffing office to make sure that the right mix of skill levels is available for the safest patient care.

Beyonce meets the HR director first who tells her that the HR department is under many employment laws, including federal, state, and institution specific. Here are some major laws that the HR director knows nurses should be aware of under the U.S. Equal Employment Opportunity Commission (EEOC):

- Title VII prohibits discrimination against race, color, religion, sex, or national origin.
- The Equal Pay Act (EPA) protects against gender-based wage discrimination.
- The Age Discrimination in Employment Act (ADEA) protects older employees against discrimination.
- Title I and V is the Americans with Disabilities Act (ADA), stating that individuals cannot be discriminated against due to disabilities.

Exercise 13-1: *Multiple-choice question*
The Age Discrimination in Employment Act (ADEA) of 1967, which protects older employees against discrimination, considers age discrimination to start at age:

    A. 40
    B. 50
    C. 55
    D. 60

eResource 13-1: To learn more about these regulations, Beyonce visits the EEOC's website: [Pathway: www.eeoc.gov → select "Employer" tab, select "Discrimination by Type" and review content related to discrimination]

Sexual harassment is also included in federal laws and each organization has policies protecting nurses from sexual harassment as well as disciplinary actions that relate to any nurse or employee who sexually harasses another person. Sexual harassment is defined as unwelcomed sexual advances, request for sexual favors, and other verbal or physical conduct of a sexual nature when it affects employment status or creates an uncomfortable or hostile work environment. The HR director gives an example to Beyonce.

Exercise 13-2: *Multiple-choice question*

Nurses have a shared kitchenette break area in an operating room suite. One of the male nurses hangs up a calendar with suggestive female pictures on it. A female nurse is offended at the pictures. What would be the best course of action?

    A. Tell the manager

    B. Report the male nurse to HR for sexual harassment

    C. Take down the calendar

    D. Tell the male nurse to take it down and why

 eResource 13-2: To learn more about laws related to sexual harassment, Beyonce returns to the EEOC's website: [Pathway: www.eeoc.gov → select "Sexual Harassment" under the "Employer" tab and review content]

Exercise 13-3: *Multiple-choice question*

A patient is getting ready for discharge at 10 a.m. and states that the evening-shift nurse asked for his email and that she wants to become better friends with him because she is attracted to him. The patient states that he wished he did not give her his email. The discharge nurse should:

    A. Instruct the patient not to answer the email

    B. Tell the nurse manager

    C. Confront the evening-shift nurse about the situation

    D. Document the conversation on an incident report

The health care industry constitutes a large portion of the sexual discrimination lawsuits filed in the United States. These suits cost the industry millions of dollars a year in settlements, lost employees, and the orientation of new employees to take their positions.

Exercise 13-4: *Select all that apply*

The best protection against sexual harassment in the workplace is to:

    ❑ Work on a unit voluntarily before accepting a job to make sure that all coworkers are nonthreatening

Answers to this chapter begin on page 179.

❑ Make sure there is sexual harassment mandatory education for all employees
❑ Research if there are clear policy statements
❑ Check the genders of the coworkers who will be on your shift
❑ Stay out of secluded areas in the workplace
❑ Ask if there is a no-tolerance policy

The HR Director discusses the hiring process with Beyonce.

Exercise 13-5: *Multiple-choice question*
The competencies required for a job are directly reflected by:
     A. The skills of the person who vacated the position
     B. The mix of the unit where the position is needed
     C. The job description that describes the work
     D. The HR person who does a skill analysis

The HR director tells Beyonce that a job will be "posted," which means an advertisement for a person will be made public either internally or externally depending on the polices of the organization.

Exercise 13-6: *Select all that apply*
Job descriptions should contain the following essential information:
❑ Title
❑ Salary
❑ Objectives
❑ List of duties
❑ Reporting lines
❑ Benefits

The HR director tells Beyonce that the hiring process is a nine-stage process.

Exercise 13-7: *Ordering*
Place the stages of the hiring process in order:
_____ Screening
_____ Precepting
_____ Staff development
_____ Advertising
_____ Orientating
_____ Position posting
_____ Performance evaluation
_____ Interviewing
_____ Selecting

Answers to this chapter begin on page 179.

Exercise 13-8: *Select all that apply*

During the screening process for employment, the following information should be obtained:

- ❏ Criminal background
- ❏ Professional references
- ❏ Drug screen
- ❏ Driving record
- ❏ Employment history
- ❏ Personal references

The HR director asks Beyonce if she would like to sit in on an interview for a job posting for a medical-surgical nurse. Beyonce accepts the offer. Before the interviewee comes in, Beyonce looks over the cover letter and résumé of the candidate that was sent to the HR department prior to the interview.

Exercise 13-9: *Ordering*

The contents of a résumé should be in the following order:

_____ References

_____ Work experience

_____ Educational achievements

_____ Objective

_____ Honors

_____ Identifying data

_____ Professional organizations

_____ Community service

Exercise 13-10: *Multiple-choice question*

The purpose of a résumé is to:

A. Describe work history
B. Provide an understanding of your career goals
C. Obtain an interview
D. Describe salary requirements

The résumé that Beyonce reviews is from a graduate nurse (GN) who will be taking her NCLEX-RN® in a few weeks. The cover letter is well-written and concise. It tells Beyonce why she is applying and briefly what skills she will bring to the organization. The résumé is also well presented.

Exercise 13-11: *Select all that apply*

Presentation of a résumé should include:

- ❏ A targeted objective
- ❏ Plain white paper
- ❏ Several fonts to enhance appearance

Answers to this chapter begin on page 179.

❑ Just one page

❑ GPA from school

❑ A statement "references furnished on request"

The HR director tells Beyonce that interviews are many times a two-step process. An HR employee interviews the candidate first and then the unit director interviews the candidate. Beyonce understands now why her clinical instructors always tell students that consider each clinical experience a job opportunity. Beyonce looks over the questions that the candidate will be asked.

Exercise 13-12: *Multiple-choice question*

In a behavioral-based interview, what question would you expect to hear?

    A. What are your 5-year career goals?

    B. What would be your ideal job?

    C. Tell me about a time you had to make a split-second choice.

    D. How would you describe yourself?

Exercise 13-13: *Select all that apply*

Questions pertaining to the following information cannot be asked at an interview:

❑ Age

❑ Reason for leaving last position

❑ Salary expectations

❑ Marital status

❑ Child care

❑ Travel distance from home

Exercise 13-14: *Multiple-choice question*

Which of the following questions by the interviewer is lawful to ask?

    A. Were you born in the United States?

    B. Does your spouse have health care coverage through his or her job?

    C. Did you receive an honorable discharge from the army?

    D. Do you currently use illegal drugs?

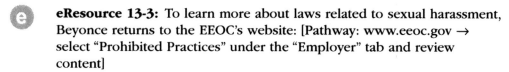 **eResource 13-3:** To learn more about laws related to sexual harassment, Beyonce returns to the EEOC's website: [Pathway: www.eeoc.gov → select "Prohibited Practices" under the "Employer" tab and review content]

The interviewee should be prepared for the interview so that all questions are answered.

Answers to this chapter begin on page 179.

Exercise 13-15: *Select all that apply*

Important tasks to complete before and during an interview include:

      ❑ Take notes

      ❑ Record the interview

      ❑ Prepare questions

      ❑ Research the organization

      ❑ Discuss the work environment

      ❑ Ask the interviewer if he or she has contacted your references

Beyonce observes several interviews being completed by the HR director. Jacob is with the nurse recruiter at a nursing school career fair and is answering questions for possible future nursing employees. The nurse recruiter is telling individuals about the organization in a positive light and is encouraging them to fill out an assessment tool, which encourages learners to rate organizations related to:

- Available unit positions and shifts
- Wages
- Benefits
- Convenience
- Vacation time
- Hospital policies related to nursing (Wittmann-Price, 2002).

Exercise 13-16: *Multiple-choice question*

The evidence informs nurses that the highest rate of burnout in a nursing position occurs due to:

      A. Benefits and wages

      B. Convenience to home and hours

      C. Vacation time

      D. Hospital policies related to nursing

One of the participants at the career fair tells the nurse recruiter that her best friend graduated and is in her first job on a medical-surgical unit working nights and is overwhelmed. The nurse recruiter tells the participant that although it is unsettling, it is a common experience.

Exercise 13-17: *Ordering*

Place the five stages of new nurse transition in order:

      _____ Exhaustion

      _____ Uses preceptor as a resource

      _____ Finds a comfort zone

      _____ Embraces policies as guides

      _____ Overwhelmed (Reddish & Kaplan, 2007)

Answers to this chapter begin on page 179.

Jacob says that this sounds like the theory he learned early on in nursing school—novice to expert. The nurse recruiter confirmed that it does fit when a graduate nurse gets a new job.

Exercise 13-18: *Matching*
Match the stage of a professional journey in Column A to the description in Column B.

Column A	Column B
A. Novice	_____ Greater than 2 to 3 years of experience, sees situation as a whole and can transfer knowledge
B. Advanced beginners	_____ No previous level of experience
C. Competent	_____ Intuitive grasp of actual impending situations
D. Proficient	_____ Some level of experience that allows the nurse to identify priorities
E. Expert	_____ Has 2 to 3 years of experience and understands the organization and what each patient needs (Benner, 1984)

The nurse recruiter also explains to Jacob that The Joint Commission (TJC) mandates that a health care facility has the right mix of competent staff to promote quality care.

Exercise 13-19: *Multiple-choice question*
Competency in an organization is ensured by:
- A. Testing employees once a year with valid test questions
- B. Orienting new employees for a set amount of time regardless of the unit
- C. Promoting professional development
- D. Returning demonstration of skills to the supervisor

After the career fair, Jacob and the nurse recruiter return to the hospital and meet up with Roxanne, who is shadowing an orientee and the preceptor on the medical-surgical unit. Roxanne asks how long the preceptorship is and the answer is that it is flexible and lasts until the graduate nurse feels ready to take an independent assignment. Roxanne asks what the difference is between preceptors and mentors.

Exercise 13-20: *Matching*
- A. A short-term relationship between an expert and novice _____ Mentoring
- B. A long-term relationship between an expert and novice _____ Precepting

Roxanne and the nurse recruiter leave the unit to go to the mandatory orientation sessions for new employees. Roxanne is interested in what content is covered in the week-long classes.

Answers to this chapter begin on page 179.

Exercise 13-21: *Select all that apply*

The nurse would expect the following topics to be covered in general orientation to a health care organization:

❑ Mission

❑ Salary

❑ Customer service

❑ Policies and procedures

❑ Health Insurance Portability and Accountability Act (HIPAA)

❑ Benefits

Many of the competencies that have to be renewed every year are done by computer program. These mandatory competencies are the nurse's responsibility to complete. Some nursing care units have competency days once or twice a year in which all new equipment is explained and skill in using them is verified. Roxanne asks the nurse recruiter if competencies are part of a nurse's yearly evaluations or performance appraisals. The nurse recruiter tells Roxanne that competency completion is a part of the evaluation but not the only element evaluated.

 eResource 13-4: Roxanne remembers that her instructor showed the class the National League for Nursing's Nursing Education Competency Model:
http://goo.gl/Pbl7M

Exercise 13-22: *Multiple-choice question*

New RN orientees should have a formal performance appraisal:

A. After the mandatory orientation week

B. After the unit orientation

C. When the preceptor says they are ready

D. After the first full year of employment

Roxanne says that she will be really nervous the first time she gets evaluated and the nurse recruiter tells her do not worry, there are ways you can prepare. First know what is on the evaluation form so that you are not surprised.

Exercise 13-23: *Multiple-choice question*

The new nurse needs further teaching when she states that during the evaluation or appraisal interview:

A. "I should write down my accomplishments right before the interview."

B. "I should accept praise and criticism when given to me."

C. "I will clarify what is expected of me if I do not understand."

D. "I will review my first set of goals and make a new set for the upcoming year."

Answers to this chapter begin on page 179.

Exercise 13-24: *Multiple-choice question*

The following issues should be discussed with the employee in the appraisal interview:

    A. Clocked in 5 minutes late twice

    B. Called in ill once on a weekend

    C. Refuses to speak to coworkers after a busy day

    D. Requests vacation a specific week each summer

Exercise 13-25: *Multiple-choice question*

After the performance appraisal or evaluation session, the new nurse should:

    A. Not sign the evaluation form unless it is agreeable

    B. Discuss the interaction with the ombudsmen

    C. Dialogue about it with other nurses to see if all staff were treated fairly

    D. Reflect on the discussion and make plans for the new year

The nurse recruiter also tells Roxanne about "clinical ladders," which is a reward system for nursing excellence. The nurse recruiter takes Roxanne to a very active same-day surgery unit to talk to some of the nurses who have applied for advancement on the clinical ladder.

 eResource 13-5: Roxanne does a quick Internet search and discovers several examples of a clinical ladder:
- Kaiser Permanente's *Nursing Pathways*: http://goo.gl/AHZkY
- Rockingham Memorial Hospital's *Clinical Ladder*: http://goo.gl/y326i

Many times the steps on the clinical ladder mimic the novice-to-expert theory. The first nurse that Roxanne asks about the clinical ladder is Keisha. Keisha describes her activities.

Exercise 13-26: *Multiple-choice question*

The highly skilled nurse in patient care who is involved in nursing unit activities and precepts and mentors new employees should be at level:

    A. Clinical Nurse I

    B. Clinical Nurse II

    C. Clinical Nurse III

    D. Clinical Nurse IV

Exercise 13-27: *Multiple-choice question*

A nurse who has exceptional experience and is recognized for knowledge and leadership, is also active in unit activities, evidence-based practice, and research, is most likely at the level of:

    A. Clinical Nurse II

    B. Clinical Nurse III

    C. Clinical Nurse IV

    D. Clinical Nurse V

Answers to this chapter begin on page 179.

Exercise 13-28: *Multiple-choice question*

A nurse who is developing and assuming responsibility is most likely at which level?

    A. Clinical Nurse I

    B. Clinical Nurse II

    C. Clinical Nurse III

    D. Clinical Nurse IV

Just as Roxanne and the nurse recruiter are discussing the clinical nurse ladder criteria, a "Code Orange" was called in the ED. Roxanne asks what that means and the nurse recruiter tells her that a Code Orange is the internal code for violent behavior. Roxanne and the nurse recruiter return to the HR department and meet the HR director, Beyonce, and Jacob and a discussion ensues. The nurse recruiter explains that a safe work environment does not only mean controls on hazardous materials but also on aggressive and violent behaviors. Keeping nurses safe is a national priority and violence occurs in hospitals frequently in one of four domains, which include:

- Violence by strangers
- Violence by patients
- Violence by coworkers
- Violence by acquaintances

 eResource 13-6: To learn more about workplace violence, Roxanne visits the Occupational Safety and Health Administration (OSHA) website: [Pathway: www.osha.gov → enter "workplace violence" into the search field → select "risk factors" as well as other content]

The group discusses the factors that place health care organizations at high risk for violence.

Exercise 13-29: *Select all that apply*

Select the factors that would place a health care organization at high risk for violence:

    ❑ Unlimited public access

    ❑ Isolated work with patients

    ❑ Sparsely filled waiting rooms

    ❑ Community work

    ❑ Discharge teaching

    ❑ High-intensity lighting in corridors

Exercise 13-30: *Multiple-choice question*

Which person is the highest risk for initiating workplace violence?

    A. A patient who is upset with his/her nursing care

    B. A family member who is insisting on seeing a patient in the intensive care unit after visiting hours

    C. A patient who is a prisoner and is being guarded

    D. A family member who is chemically impaired and visiting a patient on a medical unit

Answers to this chapter begin on page 179.

Exercise 13-31: *Select all that apply*
Warning signs that coworkers may have potential for violence include:

❑ Overconfidence

❑ Excessive talking and explaining of the situation

❑ Unkempt appearance

❑ Tardiness

❑ Carelessness and performance problems

❑ Not eating with the rest of the staff

Exercise 13-32: *Multiple-choice question*
Which visitor is the least likely to become violent in a stressful patient situation?

A. The visitor who is sitting with clenched fists

B. The visitor who is staring and pointing at the nurse

C. The visitor who is pacing

D. The visitor who is sitting quietly in the corner

The group discusses methods of diffusing potentially violent situations.

Exercise 13-33: *Select all that apply*
The following interventions are helpful to diffuse a potentially violent situation:

❑ Remove the person to a secluded room

❑ Present a calm, caring approach

❑ Use therapeutic touch

❑ Speak loudly and clearly so you are understood

❑ Do not threaten back

❑ Pay complete attention to the person

Exercise 13-34: *Ordering*
The nurse is dealing with aggressive patient behavior and the patient shouts that he is sick of not being discharged and is moving toward the door with clenched fists. What should the nurse do? Please place the appropriate steps in order:

_____ Report the behavior to the manager

_____ Move away from the patient

_____ Fill out an incident report

_____ Call security

_____ Move out of the room

Roxanne tells the HR director that she understands the steps of workplace violence prevention when dealing with patients and visitors, but is less confident about how to deal with *horizontal violence* in the workplace or violence from one employee to another. The HR director tells Roxanne, Beyonce, and Jacob that conflict management and resolution are learned skills.

Answers to this chapter begin on page 179.

Exercise 13-35: *Matching*

Match the conflict creating, management, or resolution skill in Column A to the descriptor in Column B.

Column A	Column B
A. Avoiding	_____ The decision is mutually agreed upon
B. Withholding	_____ Negotiating to reach an agreement
C. Accommodating	_____ Pretending there is no problem or issue
D. Competing	_____ Finding a solution that fits all
E. Compromising	_____ Working together respectfully
F. Confronting	_____ Taking yourself out of the situation
G. Collaborating	_____ Getting your own way
H. Bargaining	_____ Making people feel good but not addressing the issue
I. Problem solving	_____ Being forthright in approach

The HR director gives the group some examples of horizontal violence:

- Gossiping
- Not helping others
- Disrespectful nonverbal communication
- Cliques that exclude
- Withholding information
- Sabotaging others' work
- Unprofessional verbal remarks

Exercise 13-36: *Multiple-choice question*

A nursing director is abrupt and rude with a new nurse when the new nurse asks for assistance. This should be reported as:

      A. Horizontal management violence

      B. Management incivility

      C. Workplace discrimination

      D. Vertical violence

(e) **eResource 13-7:** The director gives the group two articles to read and discuss:
- *Bullying Among Nurses*: http://goo.gl/V9FuL
- *Workplace Bullying and Disruptive Behavior: What Everyone Needs to Know*: http://goo.gl/SsfGN

The group next discusses positive methods of dealing with workplace horizontal violence.

Answers to this chapter begin on page 179.

Exercise 13-37: *Select all that apply*

Positive tactics to change a culture of workplace violence include:

❑ Self-reflection

❑ Discuss it without using the word violence

❑ Encourage coworkers' verbalization about their experiences

❑ Report incidences to the manager

❑ Provide in-service on anger control

❑ Periodically analyze the culture of the workplace

The group agrees that they have a better understanding of the role of the HR department and its many functions. Information about horizontal violence, Roxanne states, is especially important because she has always heard that "nurses eat their young." The HR director assures her that this does not need to be the case if new nurses are supported correctly and advocate for themselves.

 eResource 13-8: The HR director shows the group a video that is shown to all employees as part of their orientation, *Workplace Bullying Made Simple: Bullying Prevention for the Workplace*: http://goo.gl/GkYue

Answers

Exercise 13-1: *Multiple-choice question*

The Age Discrimination in Employment Act (ADEA) of 1967, which protects older employees against discrimination, considers age discrimination to start at age:
A. **40—YES**
B. 50—NO
C. 55—NO
D. 60—NO

Exercise 13-2: *Multiple-choice question*

Nurses have a shared kitchenette break area in an operating room suite. One of the male nurses hangs up a calendar with suggestive female pictures on it. A female nurse is offended at the pictures. What would be the best course of action?
A. Tell the manager—NO, this is not the first chain of command for this infraction.
B. Report the male nurse to HR for sexual harassment—NO, this is not the first chain of command for this infraction.
C. Take down the calendar—NO, this is not addressing the issue completely.
D. **Tell the male nurse to take it down and why—YES, address it with the person first.**

Exercise 13-3: *Multiple-choice question*

A patient is getting ready for discharge at 10 a.m. and states that the evening-shift nurse asked for his email and that she wants to become better friends with him because she is attracted to him. The patient states that he wished he did not give her his email. The discharge nurse should:
A. Instruct the patient not to answer the email—NO, this is the patient's decision.
B. **Tell the nurse manager—YES, this infraction is sexual harassment that involves a patient, so it must be reported immediately.**
C. Confront the evening-shift nurse about the situation—NO, this is not your responsibility in this case because it involves a patient.
D. Document the conversation on an incident report—NO, this is not your responsibility; the manager will do this after the manager speaks with the patient.

Exercise 13-4: *Select all that apply*

The best protection against sexual harassment in the workplace is to:

☐ Work on a unit voluntarily before accepting a job to make sure that all coworkers are nonthreatening—NO, people may be on good behavior when you meet them.

☒ **Make sure there is sexual harassment mandatory education for all employees—YES**

☒ **Research if there are clear policy statements—YES**

☐ Check the genders of the coworkers who will be on your shift—NO, this should be necessary.

☒ **Stay out of secluded areas in the workplace—YES**

☒ **Ask if there is a no-tolerance policy—YES**

Exercise 13-5: *Multiple-choice question*

The competencies required for a job are directly reflected by:

A. The skills of the person who vacated the position—NO, this is not true; the person may have left because he or she did not have the skill needed.

B. The mix of the unit where the position is needed—NO, this is not true because each individual job should have a skill set.

C. **The job description that describes the work—YES, this should describe the skill set.**

D. The HR person who does a skill analysis—NO, this may be done before the job is posted.

Exercise 13-6: *Select all that apply*

Job descriptions should contain the following essential information:

☒ **Title—YES, this should be included.**

☒ **Salary—YES, this should be included, but may not have specifics.**

☒ **Objectives—YES, this should be included.**

☒ **List of duties—YES, this should be included.**

☒ **Reporting lines—YES, this should be included.**

☒ **Benefits—YES, this should be included, but may not have specifics.**

Exercise 13-7: *Ordering*

Place the stages of the hiring process in order:

___3___ Screening

___7___ Precepting

___9___ Staff development

___2___ Advertising

___6___ Orientating

___1___ Position posting

___8___ Performance evaluation

___4___ Interviewing

___5___ Selecting

Exercise 13-8: *Select all that apply*

During the screening process for employment the following information should be obtained:

☒ **Criminal background—YES**

☒ **Professional references—YES**

☒ **Drug screen—YES**

❑ Driving record—NO, only if it is necessary for the job.

☒ **Employment history—YES**

☒ **Personal references—YES**

Exercise 13-9: *Ordering*

The contents of a résumé should be in the following order:

 8 **References—YES, include names and contact information.**

 4 **Work experience—YES, in reverse chronological order.**

 3 **Educational achievements—YES, in reverse chronological order.**

 2 **Objective—YES, short clear statement starting with the word "To"**

 5 **Honors—YES, these should be highlighted.**

 1 **Identifying data—YES, up front, top center in font 12 points or greater.**

 6 **Professional organizations—YES, this shows professional accountability.**

 7 **Community service—YES, those activities that pertain to the profession of nursing.**

Exercise 13-10: *Multiple-choice question*

The purpose of a résumé is to:

 A. Describe work history—NO, this is only one part of the résumé.

 B. Provide an understanding of your career goals—NO, this is only one part of the résumé.

 C. **Obtain an interview—YES, this is the main purpose.**

 D. Describe salary requirements—NO, this should not be part of the résumé.

Exercise 13-11: *Select all that apply*

Presentation of a résumé should include:

☒ **A targeted objective—YES, it should tell the interviewer for what position you are applying.**

❑ Plain white paper—NO, it should be on thicker résumé paper if possible.

❑ Several fonts to enhance appearance—NO, one simple font, at least 12 points.

❑ Just one page—NO, this is not necessarily true.

☒ **GPA from school—YES, if it is a good GPA; if your GPA in your major is higher, use that and state your GPA in nursing.**

❑ A statement "references furnished on request"—NO, list the actual references' names and contact information.

Exercise 13-12: *Multiple-choice question*
In a behavioral-based interview, what question would you expect to hear?
  A. What are your 5-year career goals?—NO, this is done in a traditional interview.
  B. What would be your ideal job?—NO, this is done in a traditional interview.
  C. **Tell me about a time you had to make a split-second choice.—YES, this provides the interviewer with behavioral information rather than perceptive information.**
  D. How would you describe yourself?—NO, this is done in a traditional interview.

Exercise 13-13: *Select all that apply*
Questions pertaining to the following information cannot be asked at an interview:
☒ **Age—YES, this can be discrimination.**
❑ Reason for leaving last position—NO, this is acceptable.
❑ Salary expectations—NO, this is acceptable.
☒ **Marital status—YES, this and sexual preference can be discrimination.**
☒ **Child care—YES, this can be discrimination.**
❑ Travel distance from home—NO, this is acceptable.

Exercise 13-14: *Multiple-choice question*
Which of the following questions by the interviewer is lawful to ask?
  A. Were you born in the United States?—NO, this can be discrimination.
  B. Does your spouse have health care coverage through his or her job?—NO, this can be discrimination.
  C. Did you receive an honorable discharge from the army?—NO, this can be discrimination.
  D. **Do you currently use illegal drugs?—YES, you cannot ask about the past but can ask about the present.**

Exercise 13-15: *Select all that apply*
Important tasks to complete before and during an interview include:
☒ **Take notes—YES, this shows interest.**
❑ Record the interview—NO, this is inappropriate and a violation of rights if the person is unaware.
☒ **Prepare questions—YES, this shows interest.**
☒ **Research the organization—YES, this shows that you are prepared.**
☒ **Discuss the work environment—YES, this shows interest.**
❑ Ask the interviewer if he or she has contacted your references—NO, this is inappropriate.

Exercise 13-16: *Multiple-choice question*
The evidence informs nurses that the highest rate of burnout in a nursing position occurs due to:
   A. Benefits and wages—NO, this is important but not the main reason people leave a job.
   B. Convenience to home and hours—NO, this is important but not the main reason people leave a job.
   C. Vacation time—NO, this is important but not the main reason people leave a job.
   D. **Hospital policies related to nursing—YES, it is the work environment or organizational culture.**

Exercise 13-17: *Ordering*
Place the five stages of new nurse transition in order.
   __2__ Exhaustion
   __4__ Uses preceptor as a resource
   __5__ Finds a comfort zone
   __3__ Embraces policies as guides
   __1__ Overwhelmed (Reddish & Kaplan, 2007)

Exercise 13-18: *Matching*
Match the stage of a professional journey in Column A to the description in Column B.

Column A	Column B
A. Novice	__D__ Greater than 2 to 3 years of experience; sees situation as a whole and can transfer knowledge
B. Advanced beginners	__A__ No previous level of experience
C. Competent	__E__ Intuitive grasp of actual impending situations
D. Proficient	__C__ Some level of experience that allows the nurse to identify priorities
E. Expert	__B__ Has 2 to 3 years of experience and understands the organization and what each patient needs (Benner, 1984)

Exercise 13-19: *Multiple-choice question*
Competency in an organization is ensured by:
   A. Testing employees once a year with valid test questions—NO, this does not ensure competency in psychomotor skills.
   B. Orienting new employees for a set amount of time regardless of the unit—NO, different units need different orientation lengths.
   C. **Promoting professional development—YES, this ensures that staff stay up to date.**
   D. Returning demonstration of skills to the supervisor—NO, this does not ensure competency in cognitive skills.

Exercise 13-20: *Matching*
A. A short-term relationship between an expert and novice __**B**__ Mentoring
B. A long-term relationship between an expert and novice __**A**__ Precepting

Exercise 13-21: *Select all that apply*
The nurse would expect the following topics to be covered in general orientation to a health care organization:
☒ **Mission—YES, this is central to any organization.**
❑ Salary—NO, this is an individual concern.
☒ **Customer service—YES, this crosses all disciplines.**
❑ Policies and procedures—NO, this is an individual unit concern.
☒ **HIPAA—YES, this crosses all disciplines.**
☒ **Benefits—YES, this affects all full time employees.**

Exercise 13-22: *Multiple-choice question*
New RN orientees should have a formal performance appraisal:
A. After the mandatory orientation week—NO, this is too early.
B. **After the unit orientation—YES, this is usually when feedback is provided.**
C. When the preceptor says they are ready—NO, this is too subjective.
D. After the first full year of employment—NO, this does not provide formative feedback.

Exercise 13-23: *Multiple-choice question*
The new nurse needs further teaching when she states that during the evaluation or appraisal interview:
A. **"I should write down my accomplishments right before the interview."—YES, there should be advance preparation.**
B. "I should accept praise and criticism when given to me."—NO, this should be done.
C. "I will clarify what is expected of me if I do not understand."—NO, this should be done.
D. "I will review my first set of goals and make a new set for the upcoming year."—NO, this should be done.

Exercise 13-24: *Multiple-choice question*
The following issues should be discussed with the employee in the appraisal interview:
A. Clocked in 5 minutes late twice—NO, this should not be an issue unless it is a pattern.
B. Called in ill once on a weekend—NO, this should not be an issue unless it is a pattern.
C. **Refuses to speak to coworkers after a busy day—YES, this is a red flag for incivility.**
D. Requests vacation a specific week each summer—NO, this should not be an issue unless it disrupts the unit or other staff's vacations.

Exercise 13-25: *Multiple-choice question*
After the performance appraisal or evaluation session, the new nurse should:
  A. Not sign the evaluation form unless it is agreeable—NO, you can sign if it is agreeable or not—the signature indicates that you are aware; if you disagree, then write it as such.
  B. Discuss the interaction with the ombudsmen—NO, not unless there is a grievous misgiving on the evaluation that the manager will not correct.
  C. Dialogue about it with other nurses to see if all staff were treated fairly—NO, evaluations are personal information that should not be shared.
  D. **Reflect on the discussion and make plans for the new year—YES, this is the most important implication of an evaluation.**

Exercise 13-26: *Multiple-choice question*
The highly skilled nurse in patient care who is involved in nursing unit activities and precepts and mentors new employees should be at level:
  A. Clinical Nurse I—NO
  B. Clinical Nurse II—NO
  C. **Clinical Nurse III—YES**
  D. Clinical Nurse IV—NO

Exercise 13-27: *Multiple-choice question*
A nurse who has exceptional experience, is recognized for knowledge and leadership, is also active in unit activities, evidence-based practice, and research, is most likely at the level of:
  A. Clinical Nurse II—NO
  B. Clinical Nurse III—NO
  C. Clinical Nurse IV—NO
  D. **Clinical Nurse V—YES**

Exercise 13-28: *Multiple-choice question*
A nurse who is developing and assuming responsibility is most likely at which level?
  A. **Clinical Nurse I—YES**
  B. Clinical Nurse II—NO
  C. Clinical Nurse III—NO
  D. Clinical Nurse IV—NO

Exercise 13-29: *Select all that apply*
Select the factors that would place a health care organization at high risk for violence:
☒ **Unlimited public access—YES**
☒ **Isolated work with patients—YES**
☐ Sparsely filled waiting rooms—NO, crowded rooms usually precipitate violence.
☒ **Community work—YES**
☐ Discharge teaching—NO, usually information giving does not.
☐ High-intensity lighting in corridors—NO, poorly lighted corridors do.

Exercise 13-30: *Multiple-choice question*
Which person is the highest risk for initiating workplace violence?
  A. A patient who is upset with his nursing care—NO, although this may be the case, it is not the highest risk.
  B. A family member who is insisting on seeing a patient in the intensive care unit after visiting hours—NO, although this may be the case, it is not the highest risk.
  C. A patient who is a prisoner and is being guarded—NO, although this may be the case, it is not the highest risk.
  D. **A family member who is chemically impaired and visiting a patient on a medical unit—YES, drugs and alcohol always increase the risk.**

Exercise 13-31: *Select all that apply*
Warning signs that coworkers may have potential for violence include:
❑ Overconfidence—NO, this is not an indication.
❑ Excessive talking and explaining of situation—NO, this is not an indication, it is usually the nonverbal person who is at risk.
☒ **Unkempt appearance—YES**
☒ **Tardiness—YES**
☒ **Carelessness and performance problems—YES**
☒ **Not eating with the rest of the staff—YES**

Exercise 13-32: *Multiple-choice question*
Which visitor is the least likely to become violent in a stressful patient situation?
  A. The visitor who is sitting with clenched fists—NO, this person is already acting out.
  B. The visitor who is staring and pointing at the nurse—NO, this person is already acting out.
  C. The visitor who is pacing—NO, this person is already acting out.
  D. **The visitor who is sitting quietly in the corner—YES, this is not an indication.**

Exercise 13-33: *Select all that apply*
The following interventions are helpful to diffuse a potentially violent situation:
❑ Remove the person to a secluded room—NO, this places you in jeopardy.
☒ **Present a calm, caring approach—YES, this will help calm the situation.**
❑ Use therapeutic touch—NO, do not touch the person; it may infuriate him or her.
❑ Speak loudly and clearly so you are understood—NO, speak softly.
☒ **Do not threaten back—YES, this will help calm the situation.**
☒ **Pay complete attention to the person—YES, this will help calm the situation.**

Exercise 13-34: *Ordering*

The nurse is dealing with aggressive patient behavior and the patient shouts that he is sick of not being discharged and is moving toward the door with clenched fists. What should the nurse do? Please place the appropriate steps in order:

__5__ Report the behavior to the manager—YES, this is done after documentation.

__1__ Move away from the patient—YES, safety first.

__4__ Fill out an incident report—YES, document it.

__3__ Call security—YES, as soon as you can.

__2__ Move out of the room—YES, safety first.

Exercise 13-35: *Matching*

Match the conflict creating, management, or resolution skill in Column A to the descriptor in Column B.

Column A	Column B
A. Avoiding	__E__ The decision is mutually agreed upon
B. Withholding	__H__ Negotiating to reach an agreement
C. Accommodating	__A__ Pretending there is no problem or issue
D. Competing	__I__ Finding a solution that fits all
E. Compromising	__G__ Working together respectfully
F. Confronting	__B__ Taking yourself out of the situation
G. Collaborating	__D__ Getting your own way
H. Bargaining	__C__ Making people feel good but not addressing the issue
I. Problem-solving	__F__ Being forthright in approach

Exercise 13-36: *Multiple-choice question*

A nursing director is abrupt and rude with a new nurse when the new nurse asks for assistance. This should be reported as:

A. Horizontal management violence—NO, this is not the term.

B. Management incivility—NO, this is not the term.

C. Workplace discrimination—NO, this is not the term.

D. **Vertical violence—YES, this is management to staff or vice versa.**

Exercise 13-37: *Select all that apply*

Positive tactics to change a culture of workplace violence include:

☒ **Self-reflection—YES, this is most important.**

❑ Discuss it without using the word violence—NO, it needs to be discussed openly.

☒ **Encourage coworkers' verbalization about their experiences—YES, it needs to be out in the open.**

❑ Report incidences to the manager—NO, address it yourself first.

❑ Provide in-service on anger control—NO, provide it on horizontal violence specifically.

☒ **Periodically analyze the culture of the workplace—YES, this will help understand the big picture.**

14

NCLEX: Getting Ready

Unfolding Case Study #14 █ Beyonce, Jacob, and Roxanne

Finally, the last semester is coming to a close and the senior students are getting ready to take their licensure exam. To apply for the exam is a process because even though the exam is a national exam, the licensing process is done by each state. The National Council of State Boards of Nursing (NCSBN) is responsible to administer the exam and the individual state issues the LPN (LVN) or RN license.

Exercise 14-1: *Multiple-choice question*
The mission of the NCSBN is to:

    A. Regulate licensure

    B. Protect the public

    C. Protect the profession's integrity

    D. Coordinate state efforts

Exercise 14-2: *Multiple-choice question*
Most graduate nurses (GNs) apply for their license in the state:

    A. They were born

    B. Of their school

    C. Of their job

    D. Of their residence

Dr. Bennett tells them about compact state licensing. Compact states are a group of states (almost half of them) that respect each other's licensing. Dr. Bennett goes through the registration process that GNs need to do to be able to sit for their licensure exam. Registration and licensure actually consist of a three-part process:

- Registering with the state from which you would like your license
- Registering with NCSBN, which uses Pearson VUE testing company to administer the NCLEX exam

• Getting a criminal background and drug test as required by the state of licensure and registering to have it completed

Exercise 14-3: *Ordering*

Place the steps needed to register for the NCLEX in order from 1 to 6:

_____ The Board of Nursing (BON) in the state to which you applied makes the candidate eligible for the NCLEX

_____ Meet the BON eligibility requirements to take NCLEX

_____ Receive Authorization to Test (ATT) from Pearson VUE

_____ Submit application to the BON

_____ Register for the NCLEX with Pearson VUE

_____ Receive confirmation of registration from Pearson VUE

Beyonce raises her hand and asks about the number of questions on the NCLEX. Dr. Bennett explains that the NCLEX is a computerized adaptive test with a total of 265 questions. Fifteen questions are practice items that the test makers are evaluating for future tests, but the candidate taking the test does not know which 15 questions. The least amount of questions that a student can receive to pass the NCLEX is 75. A total of 6 hours is allocated for the test, which works out to be approximately 1.3 minutes for each question. If the candidate answers a question incorrectly, a question is provided that is at the same or a lower level. A candidate must stay above the passing standard to be successful. The test ends when the candidate has a score that is clearly above or clearly below the passing standard. If the candidate runs out of time, the "rule of 60" applies. This means that the candidate will be successful if the competency level for the last 60 questions was above the passing standard. Some candidates have failed the NCLEX because of "rapid guessing." Therefore, it is important to take your time in reading and answering questions. The NCLEX exam now comprises several different types of questions, including hot spots, fill-in-the-blank, drag-and-drop, audio, order-response, and select-all-that-apply or multiple-response questions. These are referred to as alternative types of questions and have been added to better assess critical thinking.

Another strategy to use in studying for the NCLEX exam is to become familiar with the organization of the test. The test plan covers the four basic categories of client needs, including:

• Safe and effective care environment

• Health promotion and maintenance

• Psychosocial integrity

• Physiological integrity

Exercise 14-4: *Multiple-choice question*

Computerized adaptive tests use the following principle:

A. Provide test questions grouped by subject

B. Alternate questions between easy and difficult

C. Start with difficult questions, then provide easier ones if needed

D. Start with easy questions, then move up to difficult

Answers to this chapter begin on page 195.

Dr. Bennett explains that the test questions are developed using Bloom's taxonomy as the mechanism of increasing the difficulty of questions.

Exercise 14-5: *Ordering*

Place the verbs used in Bloom's taxonomy in order from 1 to 6 starting with the least complex:

_____ Analyzing

_____ Applying

_____ Creating

_____ Understanding

_____ Evaluating

_____ Remembering

Beyonce says that she is nervous about the exam and Dr. Bennett gives her some general guidelines to assist in the decision-making process such as Maslow's hierarchy of needs.

Exercise 14-6: *Ordering*

Order Maslow's hierarchy of human needs from 1 to 5:

_____ Self-esteem

_____ Physiological

_____ Love and belongingness

_____ Safety

_____ Self-actualization

Dr. Bennett gives the students examples of questions based on Maslow's hierarchy of needs.

Exercise 14-7: *Multiple-choice question*

The nurse is caring for the following patients. Which patient should the nurse assess first?

A. The patient who is crying because her infant was just moved to the neonatal intensive care unit (NICU)

B. The patient who had a tubal ligation and has active bowel sounds

C. The patient who needs discharge instructions

D. The patient who had her Foley catheter removed 2 hours ago and has not voided

Dr. Bennett tells the group an additional strategy to use in analyzing NCLEX questions is to assess the negative/positive balance of the question. For a positive question, select the option that is correct; for a negative question, select the option that is incorrect. Some students put a positive or negative sign next to the stem of the question and then read each distractor, placing a positive or negative sign next to

Answers to this chapter begin on page 195.

each. The one distractor that has the same sign as the question stem is most likely the right answer.

Exercise 14-8: *Multiple-choice question*
Which statement should not be provided in a handoff report?
    A. "The patient in Room 310 has abdominal discomfort when she coughs."
    B. "The patient in 312 is reluctant to get out of bed and needs encouragement."
    C. "The patient in 314 needs discharge instructions."
    D. "The patient in 316 just sits and reads all day so needs to get up."

Therapeutic communication is one of the long-enduring basics of nursing care. As nurses, we provide therapy, not only through what we do but also what and how we communicate with patients and families. Therapeutic communication is not what you would use in everyday conversation because it is designed to be more purposeful. Therapeutic communication is nonjudgmental, direct, truthful, empathetic, and informative (Potter & Perry, 2006). Communication and documentation are among the important threads integrated throughout the NCLEX exam. Jacob asks Dr. Bennett how to schedule the exam. After candidates receive their ATT they are responsible for scheduling an appointment to test, which is usually provided within 30 days.

Exercise 14-9: *Select all that apply*
Guidelines to follow when scheduling an NCLEX exam should include:
    ❑ Reflect on the time of day that is best for you
    ❑ Print out a map that shows the way to the test center
    ❑ Study the entire day before the test
    ❑ Exercise the day before
    ❑ Set your alarm
    ❑ Go to bed early

Dr. Bennett also tells the students to eat the morning of the test and dress so they will not be too cold or too hot. Also you need a picture identification to be let into the test center.

Exercise 14-10: *Select all that apply*
Guidelines to follow for taking the NCLEX-RN® are:
    ❑ Reading the question and all answer choices before making a selection
    ❑ Making sure you understand what the question is asking
    ❑ Taking your time to be sure you have answered all questions as best as you can
    ❑ Being in charge of how you use your time by pacing yourself—avoid rapid guessing or spending too much time on any one question

Answers to this chapter begin on page 195.

❑ Wearing earplugs if you become distracted easily

❑ Not changing your answers

❑ Leaving the question blank if you do not know the answer

❑ As you answer the questions, eliminating choices that you know are incorrect

❑ Finding key words or phrases in the question that will help you choose the correct answer

❑ Being sure you are responding to the question that is being asked.

❑ Remembering that you are not expected to know everything; standardized exams have higher-level questions that will challenge the limits of your knowledge (Thompson, 2010).

Beyonce, Jacob, and Roxanne feel more confident about the exam and how to complete the registration process. They promise Dr. Bennett to email him as soon as they pass and let him know where they have gotten a job!

Answers to this chapter begin on page 195.

Exercise 14-1: *Multiple-choice question*

The mission of the NCSBN is to:

A. Regulate licensure—NO, this is a purpose but not the overall mission.

B. **Protect the public—YES**

C. Protect the profession's integrity—NO, this is a purpose but not the overall mission.

D. Coordinate state efforts—NO, this is a purpose but not the overall mission.

Exercise 14-2: *Multiple-choice question*

Most graduate nurses (GNs) apply for their license in the state:

A. They were born—NO

B. Of their school—NO

C. **Of their job—YES, where they will be working.**

D. Of their residence—NO, they can live in one state and work in another.

Exercise 14-3: *Ordering*

Place the steps needed to register for the NCLEX in order from 1 to 6:

__5__ The Board of Nursing (BON) in the state to which you applied makes the candidate eligible for the NCLEX

__2__ Meet the BON eligibility requirements to take NCLEX

__6__ Receive Authorization to Test (ATT) from Pearson VUE

__1__ Submit application to the BON

__3__ Register for the NCLEX with Pearson VUE

__4__ Receive confirmation of registration from Pearson VUE

Exercise 14-4: *Multiple-choice question*

Computerized adaptive tests use the following principle:

A. Provide test questions grouped by subject—NO

B. Alternate questions between easy and difficult—NO

C. Start with difficult questions, then provide easier ones if needed—NO

D. **Start with easy questions, then move up to difficult—YES, this is the method they work on, so the candidate answers higher level questions.**

Exercise 14-5: *Ordering*

Place the verbs used in Bloom's taxonomy in order from 1 to 6 starting with the least complex:

- __4__ Analyzing
- __3__ Applying
- __6__ Creating
- __2__ Understanding
- __5__ Evaluating
- __1__ Remembering

Exercise 14-6: *Ordering*

Order Maslow's hierarchy of human needs from 1 to 5:

- __4__ Self-esteem
- __1__ Physiological
- __3__ Love and belongingness
- __2__ Safety
- __5__ Self-actualization

Exercise 14-7: *Multiple-choice question*

The nurse is caring for the following patients. Which patient should the nurse assess first?

- A. **The patient who is crying because her infant was just moved to the NICU—YES, because there are no physiological needs in this group of patients, so psychological is next.**
- B. The patient who had a tubal ligation and has active bowel sounds—NO, no physiological need.
- C. The patient who needs discharge instructions—NO, no physiological need.
- D. The patient who had her Foley catheter removed 2 hours ago and has not voided—NO, no physiological need.

Exercise 14-8: *Multiple-choice question*

Which statement should not be provided in a handoff report? **(Negative)**

- A. "The patient in Room 310 has abdominal discomfort when she coughs."—NO, this is objective (positive).
- B. "The patient in 312 is reluctant to get out of bed and needs encouragement."—NO, this is objective (positive).
- C. "The patient in 314 needs discharge instructions."—NO, this is objective (positive).
- D. **"The patient in 316 just sits and reads all day so needs to get up."—YES, this is subjective (negative).**

Exercise 14-9: *Select all that apply*

Guidelines to follow when scheduling an NCLEX exam should include:

☒ **Reflect on the time of day that is best for you—YES, schedule the exam for the time of day when it is easiest for you to think.**

❑ Print out a map that shows the way to the test center—NO, actually take a practice drive to the test center.

❑ Study the entire day before the test—NO, relax at least half the day.

☒ **Exercise the day before—YES, this will help you to sleep.**

❑ Set your alarm—NO, set at least two alarms.

☒ **Go to bed early—YES**

Exercise 14-10: *Select all that apply*

Guidelines to follow for taking the NCLEX-RN® are:

☒ **Reading the question and all answer choices before making a selection—YES**

☒ **Making sure you understand what the question is asking—YES**

☒ **Taking your time to be sure you have answered all questions as best as you can—YES**

☒ **Being in charge of how you use your time by pacing yourself—avoid rapid guessing or spending too much time on any one question—YES**

☒ **Wearing earplugs if you become distracted easily—YES**

❑ Not changing your answers—NO, change them if you have a good reason to.

❑ Leaving the question blank if you do not know the answer—NO, leaving a question blank will not help your scoring.

☒ **As you answer the questions, eliminating choices that you know are incorrect—YES**

☒ **Finding key words or phrases in the question that will help you choose the correct answer—YES**

☒ **Being sure you are responding to the question that is being asked—YES**

☒ **Remembering that you are not expected to know everything; standardized exams have higher-level questions that will challenge the limits of your knowledge (Thompson, 2010)—YES**

References

American Nurses Credentialing Center (ANCC). (2013). *Magnet recognition program.* Retrieved from http://www.nursecredentialing.org/Magnet/ProgramOverview/New-Magnet-Model.aspx

Benner, P. (1984). *From novice to expert.* Menlo Park, CA: Addison-Wesley.

Bloom, B. S. (1956). *Taxonomy of educational objectives, handbook I: The cognitive domain.* New York: David McKay Co.

Davis, A. J., Fowler, M. D., & Aroskar, M. A. (2010). *Ethical dilemmas and nursing practice* (5th ed.). Upper Saddle River, NJ: Pearson.

Gardner, J. W. (1990). *On leadership.* New York, NY: Free Press.

Grohar-Murray, M. E., & Langan, J. (2011). *Leadership and management in nursing.* Upper Saddle River, NJ: Pearson.

Grossman, S. C., & Valigra, T. M. (2005). *The new leadership challenge.* Philadelphia: F. A. Davis.

Hoyt, R. E., Bailey, N., & Yoshihashi, A. (2012). *Health informatics: Practical guide for healthcare and information technology professionals* (5th ed.). Raleigh, NC: Lulu.com.

Institute of Medicine (IOM). (1999). *To err is human.* Retrieved from http://www.iom.edu/~/media/Files/Report%20Files/1999/To-Err-is-Human/To%20Err%20is%20Human%201999%20%20report%20brief.pdf

Kelley, R. E. (1998). In praise of followers. In W. E. Rosenbach & R. T. Taylor (Eds.), *Contemporary issues in leadership* (4th ed., pp. 96–106). Boulder, CO: Westview Press.

Kelly-Heidenthal, P., & Marthaler, M. T. (2005). *Delegation of nursing care.* Clifton Park, NJ: Thomson Delmar Learning.

Klainberg, M., & Dirschel, K. M. (2010). *Today's nursing leader.* Sudbury, MA: Jones and Bartlett.

Liker, J. (2004). *The Toyota way.* New York, NY: McGraw-Hill.

Maslow, A. (1954). *Motivation and personality.* New York, NY: Harper and Row.

Motacki, K., & Burke, K. (2011). *Nursing delegation and management of care.* St. Louis, MO: Mosby.

National Council of State Boards of Nursing (NCSBN). (2009). *NCLEX-RN Test Plan.* Chicago: Author.

Porter-O'Grady, T., & Malloch, K. (2013). *Leadership in nursing practice.* Sudbury, MA: Jones and Bartlett.

Reddish, M., & Kaplan, L. (2007). When are new graduates competent in the critical care unit? *Critical Care Quarterly, 30*(3), 199–205.

Rosenbach, W. E., & Taylor, R. L. (1998). Followership: The underappreciated dimension. In W. E. Rosenbach & R. T. Taylor (Eds.), *Contemporary issues in leadership* (4th ed., pp. 85–88). Boulder, CO: Westview Press.

Sullivan, E., & Decker, P. (1992). *Effective management in nursing* (3rd ed.). Redwood City, CA: Addison-Wesley.

Thompson, B. R. (2010). Test success. In R. A. Wittmann-Price & B. Reap Thompson (Eds.), *NCLEX-RN® EXCEL: Test success through unfolding case study review.* New York, NY: Springer Publishing Company.

Wittmann-Price, R. A. (2002). A tool to help you choose. *Advance for Nurses* (Greater Philadelphia Sept. 2).

Wittmann-Price, R. A., Anselmi, K. K., & Espinal, F. (2010, March/April). Creating opportunities for successful international student service-learning experiences. *Holistic Nursing Practice, 24*(2), 89–98. doi: 10.1097/HNP.0b013e3181d3994a

Yoder-Wise, P. S. (2011). *Leading and managing in nursing* (5th ed.). St. Louis, MO: Mosby.

Index

CPSIA information can be obtained
at www.ICGtesting.com
Printed in the USA
LVOW09s1914200117

521668LV00010B/131/P

9 780826 110381